The Agent of Trachoma

Monographs in Virology

Vol. 7

Editor: J. L. MELNICK, Houston, Tex.

S. Karger · Basel · München · Paris · London · New York · Sydney

The Agent of Trachoma

Recent Studies on the Biology, Biochemistry and Immunology of a Prokaryotic Obligate Parasite of Eukaryocytes

YECHIEL BECKER

Laboratory for Molecular Virology, Institute of Microbiology, Hebrew University-Hadassah Medical School, Jerusalem

12 figures and 5 tables

19 74

S. Karger · Basel · München · Paris · London · New York · Sydney

Monographs in Virology

Vol. 3
HOTCHIN, J. (Albany, N.Y.): Persistent and Slow Virus Infections
X + 210 p., 26 fig., 11 tab., 1971
ISBN 3-8055-1176-0

Vol. 4
NEURATH, A. ROBERT and RUBIN, BENJAMIN A. (Philadelphia, Pa.):
Viral Structural Components as Immunogens of Prophylactic Value
VI + 87 p., 11 fig., 1 cpl., 1971
ISBN 3-8055-1203-1

Vol. 5
WILDY, P. (Birmingham): Classification and Nomenclature of Viruses
VIII + 82 p., 1971
ISBN 3-8055-1196-5

Vol. 6
TINSLEY, THOMAS W. and HARRAP, KEITH A. (Oxford):
Moving Frontiers in Invertebrate Virology
VIII + 66 p., 23 fig., 3 tab., 1972
ISBN 3805-5-1464-6

S. Karger · Basel · München · Paris · London · New York · Sydney
Arnold-Böcklin-Strasse 25, CH-4011 Basel (Switzerland)

Printed in Switzerland by Buchdruckerei Merkur AG, Langenthal
ISBN 3-8055-1657-6

Contents

To the Memory of
HANS BERNKOPF (1910–1967)
Professor and Teacher of Virology

A pioneer in virus and trachoma research whose contributions to the development of research in these fields are acknowledged

Editor's Preface

Although the agent of trachoma has now been generally accepted as non-viral, it was for so long considered a virus that it seems appropriate to include this review as a Monograph in Virology. Hence, this volume should be useful not only to those working directly with the trachoma agents, but also to virologists who need an overview of the developments during the last decade which have distinguished these chlamydial agents from the viruses.

JOSEPH L. MELNICK

Preface

The opportunity to write a review on the recent developments in the research on the agent of trachoma had arisen from the invitation of Professor J. L. MELNICK to revise the review written in 1962, by the late Professor HANS BERNKOPF. As a result of marked developments in research on the immunology and biochemistry of the agent, a new review which will compile the knowledge added in the last decade seemed necessary. I have, therefore, referred mainly to studies on *Chlamydia trachomatis* which were published during the last decade. The very important studies on *Chlamydia psittaci* are beyond the scope of this monograph.

I wish to thank my colleagues, Professor I. C. MICHAELSON and Dr. B. MAYTHAR from the Department of Ophthalmology, Hadassah University Hospital, Jerusalem; Drs. Z. ZAKAY-RONES, I. SAROV, from the Department of Virology, B. GUTTER, and Y. ASHER, Y. COHEN, and H. LOKER from the Laboratory for Molecular Virology, for their continuous and enthusiastic collaboration; Professor S. E. LURIA, Department of Biology, Massachusetts Institute of Technology, Cambridge, Mass., for the critical discussions on the nature of obligate parasitism of viruses and prokaryotes in eukaryotic cells; Professor E. JAWETZ, Department of Microbiology, University of California, San Francisco, Calif., for his continuous interest and support; Dr. M. L. TARIZZO, World Health Organization, Geneva, for his continuous interest and help; Professor A. L. BARRON, on sabbatical leave from the Department of Microbiology, School of Medicine, State University of Buffalo, N.Y.; Professor H. M. JENKIN, Department of Microbiology, Hormel Institute, University of Minnesota, Austin, Minn., for the critical reading of the manuscript and for their comments; Dr. Julia Hadar for proofreading the manuscript; and my wife Miriam Becker for her continuous encouragement.

The preparation of the review was supported by a grant (No. 06-501-1.38) from the National Library of Medicine, USA, to the Israel Journal of Medical Sciences.

The research on trachoma in the author's laboratory was supported by grants from the National Institutes of Health, Bethesda, Md., USA, and the World Health Organization, Geneva, Switzerland.

The review of the literature was completed July 1972. However, some manuscripts published during 1973, while the Monograph was prepared, are also included.

I. Introduction

A. Historical Notes

Etiological studies on the trachoma agent date back to the observation by HALBERSTAEDTER and VON PROWAZEK [1907] who reported on the presence, in conjunctival cells, of inclusion bodies which contain elementary particles (designated 'Chlamydozoa' or mantle bodies). They believed, on the basis of resemblance in the morphology of the developmental cycle, that the particles in the inclusion bodies were the infectious agent of trachoma. The trachoma agent was grouped together with psittacosis and lymphogranuloma venereum into the psittacosis-lymphogranuloma-trachoma (PLT) group of organisms [THYGESON, 1962] now defined as members of the order Chlamydiales which includes one family Chlamydiaceae and two species *Chlamydia trachomatis* and *Chlamydia psittaci* (fig. 1) [PAGE, 1966, 1968, 1973]. However, 50 years elapsed from the discovery of the trachoma agent until the etiological agent of trachoma was isolated by T'ANG and his collaborators [T'ANG *et al.*, 1957, 1958], propagated in embryonated eggs, and studied with respect to its properties. Although it has been known since 1938 that the agent of trachoma and similar agents of the PLT group resembled bacteria in their sensitivity to sulfa drugs and antibacterial antibiotics, these agents were, for many years, considered as viruses. The consideration of the trachoma agent as a virus resulted in a remarkable delay in the development of trachoma research. Only after the agents of trachoma were cultivated *in vitro* was the prokaryotic nature of the agent elucidated. In 1962, BERNKOPF indicated in his review on trachoma that 'the more we learn of the nature of trachoma and related agents the less fitting the term "virus" becomes'. The indecisiveness in defining the PLT group is indicated in the constant changes in the name of the group of agents and its systematic position in the microbial world. In the 1962 symposium on the 'Biology of the Trachoma Agent', the PLT agents were regarded as viruses. In the 1966 conference on 'Trachoma and Allied Diseases', the agents were named Bedsonia. The name Chlamydia was used in the 1970 symposium on 'Tra-

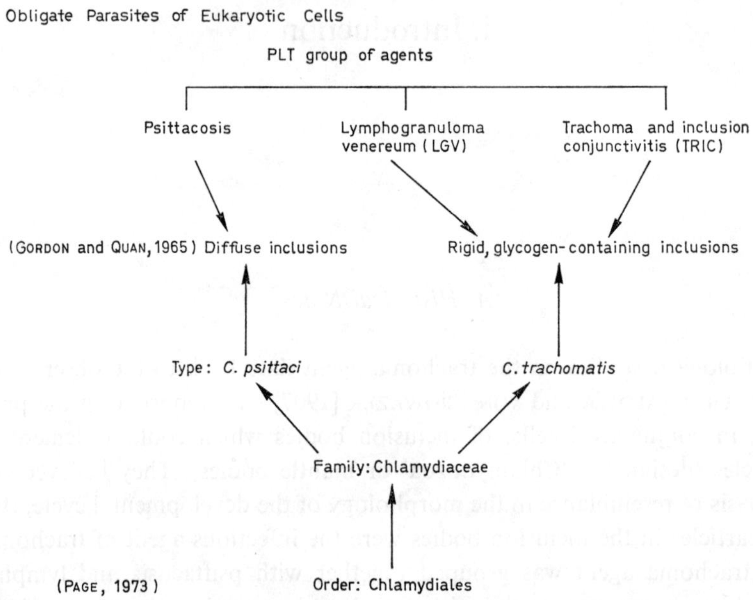

Fig. 1. The chlamydia (PLT group of agents).

choma and Related Disorders Caused by Chlamydial Agents'. However, MOULDER [1966] clearly defined the psittacosis group of agents as microorganisms which are obligate intracellular parasites of eukaryotic cells. Recent developments in the research on the molecular biology of the trachoma agent have confirmed and extended MOULDER's ideas and furthered the understanding of the chlamydial agents as prokaryotic obligate parasites. In the present review, mainly studies on *C. trachomatis* will be reviewed.

B. Recent Developments

Research on the trachoma agent has gone through several phases since the discovery by T'ANG *et al.* [1957, 1958]: the initial attempts were to isolate numerous strains of trachoma from patients in different parts of the world. This was followed by studies on the morphology and life cycle of the agent and on the effects of antibiotics on the trachoma agent. In the second phase, studies were concerned with the immunological properties of the trachoma strains and attempts were made to develop potent antitrachoma vaccines. The developments in the research on the molecular biology of microorganisms made possible studies on the molecular processes which occur during the developmental cycle of the trachoma agent. These research activities are well reflected in the scientific reports presented in three international conferences (1962, 1966 and 1970)[1] which were devoted to studies on the trachoma agent. The developments in the understanding of the chlamydia (trachoma and psittacosis agents) were reviewed by BERNKOPF [1962a, b], BIETTI and VOZZA [1963], JAWETZ [1964] and MOULDER [1966, 1971]. These reviews contain the basic information on the medical aspects of trachoma as well as the basic concepts of the chlamydial agents. The present review will deal with some of the developments in trachoma research which took place during the last decade (1962–1972)[2]. The aim of the present review is to present the current knowledge on the classification, molecular biology and immunological properties of *C. trachomatis,* the agents which cause trachoma, a disease of the human eye. These agents are members of a unique group of obligate microbial parasites of eukaryotic cells.

[1] a. The biology of the trachoma agent. Ann. N.Y. Acad. Sci *98* (1962). b. Conference on Trachoma and Allied Diseases. Amer. J. Ophthal. *63* (1967). c. NICHOLS R. L. (ed.): Trachoma and related disorders caused by chlamydial agents. Excerpta med. Int. Congr. Series, No. 223 (1971).

[2] Since the number of publications on trachoma is exceedingly high, it has become virtually impossible to quote all of them. Hence, only a relatively small number of the pertinent studies were included in the present review. A complete list of publications on trachoma is published by the Centre International de Documentation sur le Trachome, in the Revue Internationale du Trachome.

II. Definitions and Classification of the Chlamydia

A. Definitions of the Chlamydia

1. The Agents of Psittacosis, Lymphogranuloma Venereum and Trachoma (PLT) – Members of the Order Chlamydiales

In contrast to most bacterial and viral agents, whose distinct nature was easily recognized, the members of the PLT group of agents were constantly shifted from one class to another until they resumed a position on the border between viruses and bacteria [RAKE *et al.,* 1942; WEISS, 1955; MOULDER, 1966]. The indecisiveness regarding the nature of the agents and their relationship to other classes of biological entities was due to the absence of a clear definition of the group. The chlamydial agents were isolated in many laboratories during a period of 30 years from excretions of respiratory tracts (e.g. psittacosis [BEDSON and BLAND, 1932], ornithosis [POLLARD, 1947]); from genital tracts (e.g. lymphogranuloma venereum [FINDLAY *et al.,* 1938]); and from the eyes (e.g. trachoma [RAKE *et al.,* 1942; T'ANG *et al.,* 1957], inclusion conjunctivitis [FURNESS *et al.,* 1960b]). The agents isolated from humans and other vertebrates were maintained by serial transfers in the yolk sacs of developing chick embryos. Some of the agents were later adapted to growth in cultured cells *in vitro*. Numerous studies on the isolated chlamydial agents [summarized by MEYER, 1952; COX, 1953; THYGESON, 1953; WENNER, 1958; COLLIER, 1959a, b; LEPINE, 1960; BERNKOPF, 1962a, b; JAWETZ, 1964; MOULDER, 1966], as well as advancement in defining the class of viruses [LURIA, 1953; LWOFF, 1957; LWOFF and TOURNIER, 1966] and the recognition of the unique features of bacteria as a group [STANIER and VAN NIEL, 1962], led to the suggestion [PAGE, 1966, 1968] that the chlamydiae differ from Rickettsiae and constitute a specific order, Chlamydiales.

2. The Classification of the Chlamydia (PLT) Agents

Page [1966, 1968] proposed that all the agents which belong to the PLT group should be recognized as one genus: Chlamydia, Jones, Rake and Stearns, 1945. This proposal was accepted [Moulder, 1966] and in the new edition of Bergey's Manual [Page, 1973] the PLT agents were removed from the order Rickettsiales and a new order *Chlamydiales* was established [Storz and Page, 1971]. A single family, Chlamydiaceae, is recognized which contains one genus, Chlamydia, and two species: (1) *Chlamydia trachomatis* and (2) *Chlamydia psittaci*.

The following key to the species of Chlamydia was proposed [Page, 1973][3]:

(1) Forms compact microcolonies within cytoplasmic vesicles. Produces iodine-staining carbohydrate and lipid within vesicle. Growth in the yolk sac of chicken embryos is inhibited by sodium sulfadiazine (1 mg/embryo) *(Chlamydia trachomatis)*.

(2) Forms microcolonies within cytoplasmic vesicles which tend to rupture early in microcolony development, and the organisms in various stages of growth become distributed throughout the host cell cytoplasm. Does not produce iodine-staining carbohydrate or lipid in vesicles. Growth in the yolk sac of chicken embryos is not inhibited by sodium sulfadiazine (1mg/embryo) *(Chlamydia psittaci)*.

The suggestion of Page [1966] to include both *C. trachomatis* and *C. psittaci* in one genus, Chlamydia, might lead to the incorrect understanding that the members of the two species resemble each other closely enough to be placed in the same group. Studies on the molecular and biological properties led to the understanding that *C. trachomatis* and *C. psittaci* differ in many properties and are two separate and distinct entities. Therefore, it might be correct to combine Page's [1968] suggestions and part of the previous method of classification [Bergey's Manual, 6th edition; Rake, 1957]. The family Chlamydiaceae should be divided into two genera: genus I: Chlamydia with two species: (1) *Chlamydia trachomatis* and (2) *Chlamydia oculogenitalis,* and genus II: Miyagawanella (which includes the agent of psittacosis and related strains). The definitions of the two genera might be those suggested by Page [1973] to define the two chlamydia species. In the present review, the agents of trachoma and inclusion conjunctivitis (TRIC) will be named *C. trachomatis* [Page, 1966, 1968, 1973].

[3] The author is indebted to Dr. L. A. Page for a preprint of his manuscript.

All the strains of *C. trachomatis* (mainly trachoma and inclusion conjunctivitis [TRIC] agents) had been given the laboratory number of the isolate, as well as a general designation [GEAR *et al.*, 1963; HANNA, 1967]: TRIC/b/c/d/e (b = potential antigenic group; c = area of origin; d = abbreviation indicating laboratory; e = origin of clinical specimen, with further description optional: O = ocular, G = genital, T = trachoma, C = conjunctivitis, N = ophthalmia neonatorum), e.g. the G-1 strain is designated TRIC/ /WAG/MRC-1/OT. A list of isolates was prepared by the WHO reference center in San Francisco. However, the availability of immunological typing methods [WANG and GRAYSTON, 1971a, b; TREHARNE *et al.*, 1971; NICHOLS *et al.*, 1971] might provide an improved method for strain classification [GRAYSTON, 1971].

3. The Non-Viral Nature of the Chlamydia

The outdated concept that the chlamydia (PLT agents) are viruses stemmed from the description by HALBERSTAEDTER and VON PROWAZEK [1907] of the growth cycle of the trachoma agent in the conjunctival cells of infected eyes. They found that the disease was caused by small granules ('elementary bodies') which induced the formation of the inclusion bodies. The authors regarded the agent as a virus because it fulfilled all the specific criteria of viruses known at that time, namely, filterability, inclusion body formation, and obligate parasitism. Successful isolation of a psittacosis strain which formed inclusions in the cytoplasm of the infected cells was reported by BEDSON and BLAND [1932] 25 years later. The agents of psittacosis and trachoma were regarded as viruses and so were numerous agents isolated in chick embryos from infected tissues.

The modern developments in virology had led to the recognition of the differences between viruses and the 'chlamydozoa'. The viruses are considered by LURIA [1953] and by LWOFF [1957] as elements of genetic material consisting of RNA or DNA, enclosed within specific particles or virions. In the host cell, the viral genome becomes uncoated and expresses its genetic functions. Many important features of the PLT agents clearly did not fit this definition of viruses: existence of both RNA and DNA in the particles, replication by a mechanism of binary fission [LITWIN, 1959; LITWIN *et al.*, 1961; MOULDER, 1966], absence of a limiting membrane around the developing inclusions [LITWIN, 1959], the presence of enzymatic processes in the growing agents, and the formation of membranes within the developing matrix [TAJIMA *et al.*, 1957]. Rather, these characteristics of the PLT agents brought them close to the bacteria [STANIER and VAN NIEL, 1962] as suggested and demonstrated by MOULDER *et al.* [1963a, b], MOULDER [1966] and WEISS [1971].

4. The Bacterial Aspects of the Chlamydia

A definition of bacterial cells was given by STANIER and VAN NIEL [1962]: (a) prokaryotic cellular entities, which (b) reproduce by a mechanism of binary fission, (c) contain DNA and RNA, (d) possess enzymatic and metabolic activities, (e) contain cell wall material and enzymes which are concerned with the synthesis of mucopeptides, and (f) are sensitive to penicillin. The nature of the PLT agents can be discussed in the light of this definition.

The chlamydia form inclusion bodies as an integral part of their life cycle in the cytoplasm of the host cell. In the inclusions, large and small particles appear sequentially during the growth cycle. These particles contain DNA, RNA, proteins and cell wall. Ovoid particles, with a diameter of about 0.3 μm are present both extracellularly as infectious particles, and in host cell cytoplasm at the beginning and end of the developmental cycle. Larger particles, 10 μm in diameter, appear in the host cells as intermediate developmental stages; they lack infectivity, appear to be precursors of the infective particles, and reproduce by a mechanism of binary fission. Thus, although the chlamydia differ morphologically from ordinary bacteria, they resemble the latter in many properties.

B. Relationship between C. trachomatis *and* C. psittaci

The inclusion of the agents which belong to the two species into one family, Chlamydiaceae [PAGE, 1966, 1968, 1973] was based on two properties: (1) both groups of agents are obligate prokaryotic parasites of eukaryotic cells and (2) both have a common group-specific antigen. Although marked differences were noted in their biological properties, it was believed that the differences were not big enough to separate the two groups of agents. However, with the aid of molecular hybridization techniques which made possible the determination of phylogenetic relationships between organisms it became apparent [WEISS, 1971] that the members of the two groups of agents are very remote from each other.

1. Division of Chlamydia into Two Distinct Subgroups

a) Based on Biological Properties

GORDON and QUAN [1965a, b] divided the various strains of the chlamydia into two subgroups (A and B) on the basis of the biological properties of the agents. Subgroup A included the agents which formed in the infected cells compact, glycogen-containing inclusions (the agents of trachoma, inclusion conjunctivitis, lymphogranuloma venereum and mouse pneumonitis). Subgroup B included the agents which developed diffusely in the host cell cytoplasm and did not produce glycogen (the agents of human and feline pneumonitis, ornithosis, psittacosis, meningo-pneumonitis, bovine encephalomyelitis and others with similar properties).

b) Based on Susceptibility to Sulfadiazine and D-Cycloserine

LIN and MOULDER [1966] studied the properties of the members of the two subgroups of GORDON and QUAN [1965a, b] for their susceptibility to antibiotics. They found that subgroup A was homogeneous in respect to sensitivity to sulfadiazine and D-cycloserine. The members of subgroup B were resistant to sulfadiazine and much less sensitive to D-cycloserine.

c) Based on Antigenicity

The members of the two chlamydia subgroups were found to contain a group-specific antigen, which was studied by the complement fixation (CF) test [RAKE *et al.*, 1942]. Specific immunological differences between the two subgroups were distinguished by the specially prepared CF antigens and by adsorption of sera with group antigens [TERZIN *et al.*, 1964; PHILIP *et al.*, 1967]. A species-specific reaction to members of subgroup A (TRIC agents) by an indirect hemagglutination test had been reported [MOULDER *et al.*, 1963b].

d) Based on DNA Homology

KINGSBURY and WEISS [1968], WEISS *et al.* [1970] and WEISS [1971] demonstrated that DNA reassociation between *Chlamydia psittaci* and *Chlamydia trachomatis* DNAs was only 10% of the homologous reassociation reaction. The small amount of reassociation was dissolved at low temperatures, which indicated incomplete annealing. However, a marked homology and complete reassociation was obtained with single-stranded DNA molecules from any two members of either the *C. psittaci* subgroup or the *C. trachomatis* subgroup. The results indicated that the members of *C. trachomatis* were unrelated to the *C. psittaci* agents.

2. Further Subdivision of the *C. trachomatis* Agents

C. trachomatis agents were subdivided into several types on the basis of immunological differences [KATZENELSON and BERNKOPF, 1965; NICHOLS and McCOMB, 1964; BELL and McCOMB, 1967]. With the aid of the mouse toxicity prevention test [BELL and THEOBALD, 1962], ALEXANDER *et al.* [1967] were able to subdivide the TRIC agents into six immunological types. Further studies, using immunofluorescence techniques [WANG and GRAYSTON, 1970, 1971a, b; WANG, 1971], confirmed the presence of at least 6 distinct immunological types among the TRIC agents and subdivided them into two major groups: (a) the immunological types A, B, Ba and C, isolated from the eyes of trachoma patients, and (b) the immunological types D, E and F, which were isolated from the genital tracts of humans [WANG and GRAYSTON, 1971a, b, c]. The agents which were typed as A, B, Ba and C are the agents which cause classical trachoma in human eyes, while the immunological types D, E and F are not trachoma agents but genital TRIC agents (table I). This definition was not always possible, and COLLIER [1971] indicated that a strain with a D prototype was isolated from a case of classical trachoma. Utilizing an indirect immunofluorescence test to detect and quantitate serum antibodies to the six antigenic types of *C. trachomatis,* it was found that different groups of patients suffering from acute or chronic TRIC infections differed in the type of the infecting agent [HANNA *et al.,* 1972].

WANG *et al.* [1973] reported on the characterization of three additional antigenic types (G, H, I). Type G was related to type F and appeared to be an immunological bridge between type F and types B, Ba, D, E and the LGV-related types. Types H and I were completely unique immunologically, and strains of the new types had been isolated almost entirely from the human genital tract.

C. Evolution of the Chlamydial Agents

1. Evolutionary Relationship between *C. trachomatis* and *C. psittaci*

MOULDER [1966] indicated that subgroup A *(C. trachomatis)* of the PLT group of agents was a highly uniform collection of organisms, which suggested a comparatively recent common origin. The members of subgroup A had two synthetic abilities (synthesis of glycogen and folates) that the members of subgroup B *(C. psittaci)* lacked. Therefore, the latter organisms

Table I. Origin of 165 TRIC strains typed by the mouse toxicity prevention test and/or the micro-immunofluorescence test

Origin	TRIC type							Number of strains tested
	C	A	B	Ba	D	E	F	
Geographical								
Australia			2					2
India	15		1					16
China	1							1
Taiwan	45		14			3	8	70
Japan	1					1		2
Iran	8		2					10
Saudi Arabia	2	3	2					7
Egypt		1						1
Ethiopia		3		3				6
Gambia		1	3		1		2	7
Portugal		2						2
U.K.			1[3]		1	2	3	7
Denmark					2	5	4	11
Canada	1[1]							1
USA	1[2]			4	4	10	3	22
Clinical								
Ocular trachoma	74	10	25	7	3[4]	1[5]	1[6]	121
Ocular: IC, PKC	0	0	0	0	1	12	5	18
Genital: Cx, Ureth.	0	0	0	0	4	8	14	26
Total	74	10	25	7	8	21	20	165

From Wang and Grayston [1971c; p. 31].
[1] UW-1.
[2] AP-1.
[3] Lt-1.
[4] G-1 Pima DK-10.
[5] Bour.
[6] DK-17.

Table II. Evolution of *C. trachomatis*

Ancestor	LGV	Genital	Intermediate		Ocular
? →	I, II and III →	D, E and F →	Ba →	B →	A and C

After Wang and Grayston [1971a, b, c].

could be regarded as closer to the ancestor. The DNA homology studies reported by WEISS *et al.* [1970] and WEISS [1971] minimized the possibility of any evolutionary relationship between *C. trachomatis* and *C. psittaci* [WEISS, 1971]. WEISS suggested that the common ancestor of *C. trachomatis* and *C. psittaci* must be quite remote to account for the differences in the DNA sequences and the lack of DNA homology between the two subgroups. In the present review, attention will be focused on *C. trachomatis.* Studies on *C. psittaci* were recently summarized by STORZ [1971].

2. Evolution of *C. trachomatis* Strains

WANG and GRAYSTON [1971a, b, c], on the basis of the one-way cross-reactions which were demonstrated between certain *C. trachomatis* types, suggested the relationship of one type to another. They assumed that the lymphogranuloma venereum (LGV) strains were the earliest strains historically. Genital TRIC agents types D and E were derived from the LGV strains. One strain (designated Ba) represented a bridge from genital TRIC agents to ocular trachoma strains. The B strain represented a further change from the Ba strain, losing the close immunological relationship to genital TRIC and LGV strains. WANG and GRAYSTON [1971a, b, c] also suggested that the ocular trachoma strains were historically more recent than the genital strains, which in turn are more recent than LGV (table II).

These studies led to the conclusion that except for the common antigen there are marked differences between *C. trachomatis* and *C. psittaci* agents. However, if the studies by WANG and GRAYSTON [1971a, b, c] and WANG *et al.* [1973] are confirmed, then the evolutionary trait for *C. trachomatis* agents might be established. The molecular differences between LGV and the trachoma agent are not yet known, and further studies on these aspects are needed to establish the biochemistry of chlamydia evolution.

III. Isolation and Propagation of TRIC and Related Agents

A. Isolation of TRIC Agents from the Conjunctivae of Trachoma Patients

1. Difficulties in the Diagnosis of Trachoma and Inclusion Conjunctivitis

The diagnosis of trachoma is based on the presence of specific conjunctival and corneal signs. However, a differentiation between an infection in the eye caused by the agent of trachoma or by the agent of inclusion conjunctivitis is quite difficult [THYGESON, 1967]. The usual course of trachoma infection leads to a chronic infection characterized by the formation of follicles, papillar hyperplasia, pannus and scars. Inclusion conjunctivitis heals spontaneously without scars and pannus [THYGESON, 1967]. These features of inclusion conjunctivitis are typical of infections in the eyes of newborns (also named inclusion blennorrhea or inclusion ophthalmia neonatorum). However, DAWSON and SCHACHTER [1967] indicated that the identification of the agent of trachoma and inclusion conjunctivitis as distinct species is based on clinical differences between the two eye diseases and that there is a spectrum of the clinical diseases. In contrast, the reaction of adults' eyes to the agent of inclusion conjunctivitis results in trachoma-like severe disease with scars and pannus [JONES, 1964; JONES and COLLIER, 1962]. These authors indicated that one strain (LB4), which was isolated from a case of neonatal inclusion blennorrhea, was capable of producing trachoma symptoms in the adult eye.

In contrast to the difficulty in the clinical differentiation between trachoma and inclusion conjunctivitis, THYGESON [1967] indicated that lymphogranuloma venereum (LGV) is not related to the TRIC agent clinically. LGV has an affinity for lymph vessels, producing lymph blockage and buboes not found in trachoma or inclusion conjunctivitis.

The difficulties in distinguishing between TRIC infections of the eyes were reflected in misidentification of the various chlamydial agents isolated from patients who were diagnosed as trachoma on the basis of the clinical appearance of the disease in the eyes. Thus, both trachoma and inclusion conjunctivitis agents were isolated from patients who were diagnosed as trachoma patients. Hence, the immunological typing of the isolated trachoma strains is essential for establishing the true nature of the agents.

2. Isolation of TRIC Agents in the Yolk Sac of Embryonated Eggs

a) Studies by T'ANG *and Collaborators*

The successful isolation of three agents (designated TE8, TE55 and TE66, according to the experiment number) from patients with active trachoma stage 2 was achieved by T'ANG *et al.* [1957]. Using ophthalmological swabs, the upper fornix and palpebral conjunctiva were rubbed; the swabs were then soaked in brothsaline. From the material which was treated with streptomycin, 1 strain (TE 66) was isolated in 5 experiments; after treatment with penicillin and streptomycin, 2 strains (TE8 and TE55) were isolated in 29 experiments by inoculation into the yolk sac of chick embryos. Infection of monkeys with two of the isolated strains (TE8 and TE55) resulted in the development of follicles in the monkeys' eyes after an incubation period of 7–16 days. Inoculation of 1- to 2-day-old mice intracerebrally with TE8 strain and serial intracerebral passages with brain material gave negative results, indicating that mice were refractory to the agent.

Further studies from T'ANG *et al.* [1958] led to a more efficient isolation of trachoma strains (9 out of 22 specimens). The new isolates resembled the trachoma strains previously obtained. Because of the important role that the Chinese strain TE55 had in the development of the research on the trachoma agent, special attention will be given to the studies carried out with this particular strain.

b) Further Isolations of Agents from the Conjunctivae of Trachoma Patients

Since the reports of T'ANG *et al.* [1957, 1958] on the isolation of trachoma agent and the confirmation of their findings by COLLIER and SOWA [1958], many chlamydia agents have been recovered in many laboratories [reviewed by BERNKOPF, 1962, and DAROUGAR and JONES, 1971]. The agents were isolated by inoculation into the yolk sacs of chick embryos and cell cultures of materials obtained from conjunctival scrapings [COLLIER, 1959a, b; HANNA *et al.*, 1959; JONES *et al.*, 1959; BERNKOPF *et al.*, 1959; PERRET and MANN,

1960; HANNA *et al.,* 1960; TARIZZO, 1961; HANNA, 1962; MITSUI *et al.,* 1961; MURRAY *et al.,* 1962; MORDHORST, 1964, 1965a, b, 1967a; SOWA *et al.,* 1965; TAMURA, 1964b; DAWSON and SCHACHTER, 1967; GORDON *et al.,* 1969]. Successful isolations of trachoma strains were also obtained from the eyes of trachoma patients by swabbing the conjunctiva and inoculating the material into embryonated eggs [T'ANG *et al.*, 1957, 1958; COLLIER and SOWA, 1958; COLLIER *et al.,* 1958; GEAR *et al.,* 1967; DAROUGAR and JONES, 1971].

c) Factors Affecting the Isolation of Trachoma Strains

The use of chick embryos for the isolation of TRIC agents from trachomatous eyes depended on the susceptibility of the embryos to the agents. JAWETZ [1962a] observed that at unexpected times the embryonated eggs became insusceptible to TRIC agents. The reason for this unexpected change was not determined. Therefore, in order to obtain an independent method for the isolation and propagation of the trachoma agent, a different method was needed.

B. Direct Isolation of TRIC Agents in Cultured Cells

1. The Use of McCoy Cells for the Isolation of the Trachoma Agents

GORDON *et al.* [1963] compared the usefulness of McCoy cell cultures (human synovial cell line), for direct isolation of TRIC agents, to that of embryonated eggs. They were able to detect TRIC infection in infected cell cultures within 48 h after inoculation, while in embryonated eggs several days were needed. Further studies [GORDON and QUAN, 1965b] demonstrated that TRIC agents can be isolated directly in irradiated McCoy cells, which were found to be more sensitive than unirradiated ones [GORDON *et al.*, 1967]. The cell-culture grown trachoma strains retained their immunological specificity on passage *in vitro*, and the intracellular inclusions reacted only with the homologous type-specific antiserum [GORDON *et al.*, 1971]. Usually, the infectious particles were centrifuged onto the cell monolayer to facilitate infection. It was also found [ROTA and NICHOLS, 1971] that pretreatment of McCoy cells with DEAE-dextran increased the number of cells infected with the trachoma agent. DAROUGAR *et al.* [1971a, b] demonstrated that the isolation of TRIC agents in irradiated McCoy cells is the diagnostic method of choice (fig. 2).

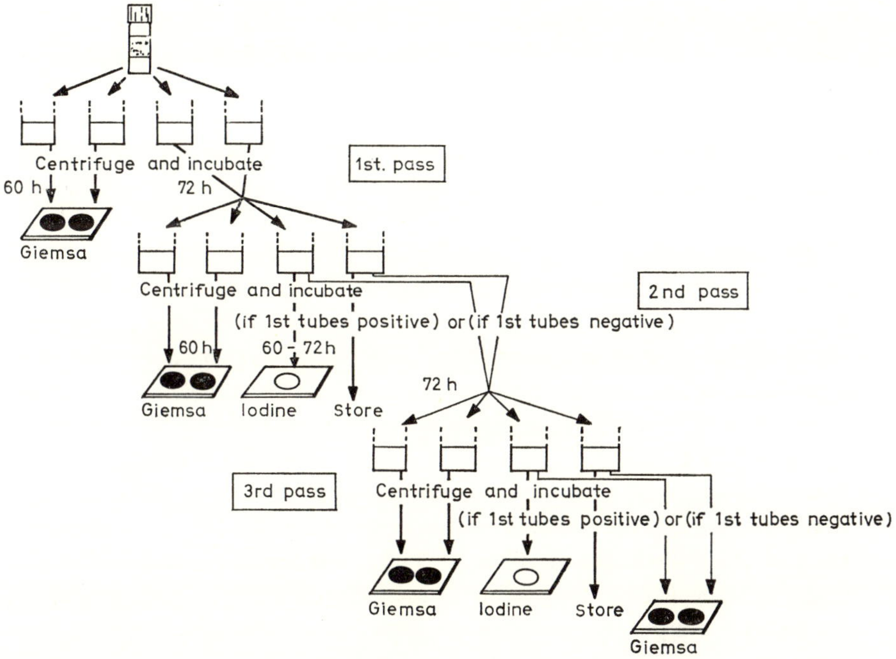

Fig. 2. Standard three-passage technique of irradiated McCoy cell culture for isolation of Chlamydia. From DAROUGAR *et al.* [1971a, p. 66].

2. Isolations of TRIC Agents from Human Disorders

a) Isolation of Trachoma Strains from the Urogenital Tract and the Rectum

The suggestion that the agent of inclusion conjunctivitis was spread primarily through the genital tract by infecting newborns at birth was originated by LINDNER [1910]. JONES *et al.* [1965] reported that adults with TRIC agent infections of the genital tract might have ocular syndromes. The development of techniques for the isolation and propagation of TRIC agents made possible the study of the genital *C. trachomatis* agents.

MORDHORST [1967a, b], DAWSON and SCHACHTER [1967], and HOLT *et al.* [1967] isolated TRIC agents from the human genital tract. MORDHORST [1967a, b] also demonstrated that young adults with trachoma also had urethritis or vulvovaginitis from which TRIC agents were isolated. DUNLOP *et al.* [1971a, b] reported on the isolation of chlamydiae from the urethra of patients with non-gonococcal urethritis, as well as on the isolation of chlamydial agents from rectal material from patients without evidence of lymphogranuloma venereum. Similar results were reported by PHILIP *et al.* [1971]. Most of the agents were isolated in irradiated McCoy cells [GORDON and QUAN, 1971]. KUO *et al.* [1972b] reported that DEAE-dextran-treated HeLa cells were as sensitive as irradiated McCoy cells for the primary isolation of genital TRIC agents.

b) Isolation of Chlamydia from LGV and Other Human Disorders

SCHACHTER (1967a) reported the isolation of chlamydial agents from (1) a patient with clinical lymphogranuloma venereum, (2) 8 out of 59 patients with arthritis (6 of these 8 patients had Reiter's syndrome. Intracamera inoculation of a chlamydial agent recovered from the synovial membrane of a patient with Reiter's syndrome produced corneal changes in the eyes of rabbits [OSTLER *et al.*, 1970]), and (3) in 4 out of 22 instances chlamydia were obtained from expelled fetuses [SCHACHTER, 1967b]. FOY *et al.* [1967] isolated TRIC agents from the cervix of pregnant women. JONES [1972] summarized the studies on the isolation of genital TRIC agents and concluded that the findings supported the suggestion that sexual transmission with genital to eye transfer is a possible factor in the spread of eye diseases.

C. Growth of C. trachomatis *in Cultured Tissues*

1. Explants of Chick Embryos

GORDON *et al.* [1960] were able to cultivate *C. trachomatis* agents *in vitro* in explants of the entodermal layer of 4-day-old chick embryos. Infection was confined to a minority of the cells, and it was difficult to obtain more than one cycle of multiplication.

2. Adaptation of *C. trachomatis* Agents to Growth in Conjunctival Cells *in vitro*

Organ cultures of rhesus monkey conjunctivae supported the growth of *C. trachomatis* [BARRON *et al.*, 1971]. Primary cultures of rabbit corneal endothelial cells were found to support growth of the T'ang strain of the trachoma agent [OH *et al.*, 1967].

3. Adaptation of Trachoma to Mouse Macrophages

Macrophages were maintained for several days *in vitro* and infected with trachoma agent [CASAZZA *et al.*, 1969; TAVERNE and BLYTH, 1971]. The two groups agree that the macrophages adsorbed the elementary bodies; CASAZZA *et al.* [1969] reported that the agent reproduced in the macrophages while TAVERNE and BLYTH [1971] could not demonstrate any e.b. development. TRIC agents also had a toxic effect on freshly seeded macrophages [TAVERNE and BLYTH, 1971].

4. Continuous Propagation of Chlamydia in Cell Lines

POLLARD *et al.* [1960a], BERNKOPF *et al.* [1960], and FURNESS *et al.* [1960b] reported the successful cultivation of several *C. trachomatis* agents in cell cultures *in vitro*. These studies made possible the investigations on the growth cycle and biochemistry of *C. trachomatis*.

The *in vitro*-propagated trachoma agents retained their pathogenicity to the human eye, causing mild inflammation and a typical course of disease [BERNKOPF *et al.*, 1964] which was self-limiting. MITSUI *et al.* [1964b, 1967] and JENKIN [1966] had found that the trachoma agent propagated in HeLa cells retained its pathogenicity to monkeys.

Most of the agents could be propagated only for a limited number of passages [BERNKOPF, 1962]. The T'ang strain of trachoma (TE55) which was adapted by BERNKOPF *et al.* [1960] to growth in FL cells had the ability to continuously propagate in the FL cells. The exact nature of this strain, however, is still questionable [WANG, 1971].

5. Enhancement of Trachoma Agent Infectivity by DEAE-Dextran

KUO *et al.* [1972a] demonstrated that pretreatment of HeLa-229 monolayers by washing with DEAE-dextran prior to inoculation of the TRIC agent resulted in an enhanced infectivity, as shown by a tenfold increase in the infective progeny. No enhancement was found when LGV agents were studied by the same technique.

D. Properties of the T'ang (TE55) Strain

One of the first strains of *Chlamydia trachomatis* isolated by T'ANG *et al.* [1957] in Peking was the TE55 strain which was sent to Dr. L. COLLIER and distributed to several laboratories. The TE55 strain was since propagated in various tissues and cell cultures and during subsequent years conflicting reports were published on its properties. Since this strain was used as a model for *C. trachomatis* agents, the properties of this agent will be analyzed to determine when and how changes in its properties appeared.

1. Early Passages of the TE55 Strain in Chick Embryos

Freeze-dried samples of two Chinese strains (TE8 and TE55) were brought from Peking (September 1957) to Dr. L. H. COLLIER's laboratory at the Lister Institute, London. The strains were revived by passage in the yolk sacs of 8-day-old embryonated eggs incubated at 35 °C. After three egg passages, the TE55 strain caused follicles in the upper fornix of the inoculated eyes of two monkeys. Cytoplasmic inclusions were occasionally found in scrapings from the infected conjunctiva, but never typical ones [COLLIER and SOWA, 1958]. The TE55 strain was distributed to other laboratories.

2. Adaptation of TE55 to Growth in Cell Cultures

The TE55 strain was received in BERNKOPF's laboratory in Jerusalem after an unknown number of passages in embryonated eggs, which were carried out abroad [BERNKOPF, 1959]. The author noted that the TE55 strain multiplied more intensely in the yolk sac than a local trachoma isolate and killed the chick embryos within 4–6 days. The TE55 trachoma strain killed mice by intracerebral inoculation. The same TE55 strain was adapted to growth in FL cell cultures [BERNKOPF *et al.*, 1960]. The trachoma agent developed inclusion bodies in the cytoplasm of the host cells, which, at the end of the growth cycle, contained elementary bodies infectious to chick embryos. At the sixth passage level in FL cell cultures, the TE55 strain was infectious to a human volunteer after instillation in the eye. The clinical symptoms which resulted were of a mild trachoma infection, with a number of follicles on the 9th day. The TE55 strain has been continuously propagated in FL cell cultures ever since. There were no changes in the time course of the agent's developmental cycle (48 h) [Bernkopf *et al.*, 1962a]. Also, the time when glycogen was synthesized in the inclusion bodies has remained unchanged during the last 10 years. In respect to killing embryonated eggs by yolk sac inoculation, death of embryos was attained 4–6 days after inoculation of a large dose of elementary bodies (10^4–10^5 egg infective units) [Becker *et al.*, 1969a, b]. Therefore, we assume that the TE 55 strain retained its original characteristics, in agreement with Reeve and Taverne [1967a, b].

3. Properties of the TE 55 Strain Propagated in Other Cell Lines

Collier [1962] reported that in April 1959 it was noted that the TE 55 strain, which had been propagated in mouse brain [Hurst and Reeve, 1960], formed cytoplasmic inclusions in monkey kidney cells. Soon after, similar inclusions were induced in rabbit embryo kidney and HeLa cells and later on the agent was grown in cell cultures seeded with infected yolk sac material [Collier, 1962]. The TE 55 strain used by Pollard and Tanami [1962], also obtained from Dr. L. H. Collier, showed different properties than the original TE 55 strain: (1) Pollard's TE 55 strain killed chick embryos earlier than another strain (SA-2) and (2) an enhanced form was propagated in embryonated eggs. However, the authors indicated that the T'ang trachoma strain, as received from Dr. Collier, propagated in FL cells at a slower rate than the enhanced form, and the inclusions resembled those of the TRIC agent. However, the enhanced strain isolated by Pollard and Tanami [1962] grew diffusely in the infected cell, a property of *C. psittaci* strains.

4. Propagation of TE 55 in Mice

Hurst and Reeve [1960] propagated the agents of trachoma, inclusion blennorrhea and lymphogranuloma in mice. From this study it was found that the G 1 and G 17 strains of trachoma could not be passaged in mouse brain while the LB 1 strain of inclusion blennorrhea was propagated. At the same time, two LGV strains (the established JH strain and a recent isolate) were also propagated in mouse brain. On intracerebral passage in mice these two agents behaved similarly to the T'ang strain and produced inclusion bodies in cell cultures. However, the authors indicated that the agents were handled in different isolation units by different personnel.

5. Development of Fast Killing (f) Strains of TE 55 and Related Agents

REEVE and TAVERNE [1963, 1967a, b] observed that during subsequent passages in the chick embryos three strains (LB 1, LB 4 and Bour) changed their behavior, killing embryos faster and acquiring the ability to form inclusions in HeLa cells. In contrast, the strains G 1 and G 17 (isolated from trachoma patients in Gambia) killed the embryos 3–4 days later than the strains SA 2, LB 1, TE 55 and LGV, which killed embryos quickly, the majority of embryos dying on the 5th day. Nevertheless, the agents (including TE 55) which killed embryos at 5 days after inoculation, were not markedly different from the original TE 55 strain, which killed chick embryos during a period ranging from 5 to 9 days. The TE 55 strain of REEVE and TAVERNE [1963] was not a fast-growing strain as compared to the original TE 55 strain, and additional studies [REEVE and TAVERNE, 1967a, b] demonstrated that 'fast killing' (f) strains of various TRIC agents also developed. The 'f' TE 55 was only slightly pathogenic for monkeys [REEVE and TAVERNE, 1967a, b].

Table III. Micro-IF cross-test of LGV and 'fast' strains

Antisera	Antigens										Homologous titers
	440	434	JH	LB-1	LB-1 f	LB-4 f	Bour f	SA-2 f	PK-2 f	347 F	
440 (I)[1]	100	13[2]	25	25		25	13	25	25	13	128–256
434 (II)	13	100	100	100	100	100	100	100	100	13	64–128
JH (II)	25	100	100	100	100	100	100	100	100	13	512–1,024
LB-1	25	100	100	100	100	100	100	100	100	25	512
LB-1 f		50		100	100	100	100	100	100		1,024–2,048
LB-4 f	25	100	100	100	100	100	100	100	100	6	512
Bour f	13	100	100	100	100	100	100	100	100	25	512–1,024
SA-2 f	13	100		100	100	100	100	100	100	13	1,024–2,048
PK-2 f	13	100	100	100	100	100	100	100	100	13	512–1,024
347 F (III)	13	13	13	13	13	13	6	25	25	100	1,024

From WANG and GRAYSTON [1971 a].

[1] LGV strain type I, type II, or type III in parentheses.

[2] Percent of homologous titer.

6. Antigenic Differences of TE 55 Strains

REEVE and TAVERNE [1967a, b] suggested a possible antigenic change in the fast killing strains. Further studies by GRAHAM [1967] demonstrated that all 'f' strains show complete cross-immunization against each other but 'slow killing' ('s') strains were protective in the homologous systems only. WANG and GRAYSTON [1971 a], using the micro-immunofluorescence test, demonstrated that all the 'f' strains, derived from various strains of the trachoma agent, were antigenically identical with the JH strain of lymphogranuloma venereum (LGV) (table III). However, these authors clearly distinguish between the 'slow killing' strain of TE 55, which was designated TRIC/China/Peking-2/OT (abbreviated to PK-2) and typed as *C. trachomatis* agent, and the 'fast killing' strain which was found to be identical to the JH strain of LGV.

These studies [WANG and GRAYSTON, 1971a] indicated that 'f' strains, which were obtained after 1959 and behaved as 'fast killing' strains, might have arisen due to contamination with the JH strain of LGV, while the 's' strains might have retained the characteristics of the original TE 55 strain.

7. Antigenic Properties of the T'ang TE 55 Strain

This strain was obtained from Dr. L. COLLIER by Dr. H. BERNKOPF and was propagated in the yolk sacs of embryonated eggs. Initial experiments by BERNKOPF *et al.* [1964] on the pathogenicity of the agent in human eyes revealed that a mild trachoma infection resulted upon infection of a volunteer. It was therefore concluded that the T'ang (TE 55) strain can cause an eye disease similar to trachoma. However, this strain differed from the other trachoma agents which were isolated from active trachoma infections in human eyes. The latter strains were propagated in the yolk sacs of embryonated eggs but did not propagate in cell cultures *in vitro*. The T'ang strain can be propagated in cell cultures without difficulty.

Recent studies by WANG [personal commun.] on the antigenicity of the TE 55 strain from our laboratory revealed that it resembled the TE 55 strain from Dr. COLLIER's laboratory. However, laboratory contamination with a lymphogranuloma venereum strain could be ruled out as such strains were not propagated in the laboratory at the time. We concluded that the ability of the TE55 strain to cause trachoma in a volunteer might indicate that it is a potent agent of trachoma. This strain, which has the ability to develop in cell cultures was used as a model system for studies on the molecular biology of *C. trachomatis* agents.

IV. The Biology of the Trachoma Agent

The trachoma agent, an obligate prokaryotic parasite of eukaryocytes, initiates its developmental cycle after entry into the cytoplasm of a sensitive host cell. Its ability to reproduce is controlled by the genetic apparatus of the agent and the microenvironment in the host cell cytoplasm. The nutritional requirements and the mode of reproduction will be discussed.

A. The Developmental Cycle

1. The Interaction of e.b. with Host Cells

Addition of a suspension of *C. trachomatis* e.b. to monolayers of cultured cells resulted in the adsorption of the e.b. to the cell membrane. FURNESS *et al.* [1962] treated e.b. at 56 °C prior to infection and found that the inactivated e.b. were retained on the cell membrane for a period of 6 h. FURNESS and FRASER [1962] found that the e.b. also interacted with cells at 30 °C but further development of e.b. was arrested. A quantitative analysis of the interaction of *C. trachomatis* (TE 55) e.b. demonstrated that the e.b. interacted with the FL cell membranes in a manner which resembled virus attachment [BECKER *et al.*, 1969b]. The interaction was rapid, starting immediately after the addition of the e.b. to the cell cultures and reaching maximum after 3 h. Heparin, a negatively charged polysaccharide, caused the release of the e.b. which attached to the cells, indicating that the interaction of e.b. with the cell membrane was electrostatic in nature. It was also demonstrated that subsequently the e.b. were engulfed into the host cell cytoplasm. Metabolic processes in the e.b. started 3 h after attachment to the cells. FRIIS [1972] demonstrated that *C. psittaci* e.b. enter the host cell by an act of phagocytosis by the host cell, independent of an adsorption stage.

2. Site of Development in the Infected Cell

The e.b. present in the cytoplasm of infected cells were detected by staining with Giemsa or acridine orange stains [FURNESS *et al.*, 1962; POLLARD and TANAMI, 1962; BERNKOPF *et al.*, 1962a; COLLIER, 1962]. These techniques demonstrated that the e.b. of the agents of inclusion blennorrhea or trachoma were first observed adjacent to the cell nuclei at 3 h after infection [FURNESS *et al.*, 1962; BERNKOPF *et al.*, 1962a].

3. The Biological Activity of Trachoma Elementary Bodies – Determination of Infectivity

The trachoma e.b. are the infectious stage of the *C. trachomatis* developmental cycle. To determine the infectivity of the e.b., the latter were titrated either in embryonated eggs or in cultured cells.

a) Titration in Embryonated Eggs

To quantitate the e.b. content in a preparation, tenfold dilutions of the infected yolk sac material were inoculated into embryonated eggs. After incubation for 6 or more days at 35 °C, the infected eggs were screened for the death of the embryos and the presence of elementary bodies in stained yolk material. JAWETZ [1964] indicated that (a) the egg infective dose (EID_{50}) had no fixed relationship to the egg lethal dose (ELD_{50}) and (b) with many adapted strains the EID_{50} is threefold smaller than the ELD_{50}.

b) Titration in Cultured Cells

FURNESS *et al.* [1960a] determined the infectivity of trachoma e.b. by infecting cultured cells. The infected cells were stained at the end of the agent's growth cycle, the number of inclusions was determined microscopically, and the titer was calculated.

BERNKOPF [1967] developed a plaque assay for the titration of the trachoma agent (TE 55 strain). The infected BSC_1 monolayers were overlayed with agar and incubated in a CO_2 incubator for 6 days until plaques were formed due to the spread of the e.b. from the initially infected cells to the neighboring cells. The cultures were stained with neutral red and the plaques were counted. A linear relationship existed between the number of plaques and the concentration of e.b. in the preparation.

4. Stages of the Developmental Cycle

The growth cycle of the trachoma agent consisted of three major stages: (a) attachment and penetration of the e.b. into the host cell cytoplasm which was associated with a loss in infectivity, (b) development of inclusion bodies (no infectious e.b. could be detected in the infected cells) and (c) the synthesis of the e.b. progeny which was associated with an exponential increase in infectivity. The growth curves of inclusion blennorrhea in HeLa cell monolayers [FURNESS *et al.*, 1962; COLLIER, 1962] and the trachoma agent (TE55) in FL cells [BERNKOPF and MASHIAH, 1962; BERNKOPF *et al.*, 1962a; BECKER and ZAKAY-RONES, 1969] were reported (fig. 3). The phases of the growth cycle resembled the growth cycle of the meningopneumonitis agent [HIGASHI *et al.*, 1962]. It was repeatedly demonstrated that the second phase of the developmental cycle, during which infectivity could not be demonstrated, took place during the initial 24 h after infection. The third phase, during which infectivity gradually increased, occurred during the subsequent 24 h [BERNKOPF *et al.*, 1962a]. In recent experiments, a somewhat shorter growth cycle was found with the TE55 strain [BECKER and ZAKAY-RONES, 1969].

It was assumed that the decline in infectivity of the e.b. after entering

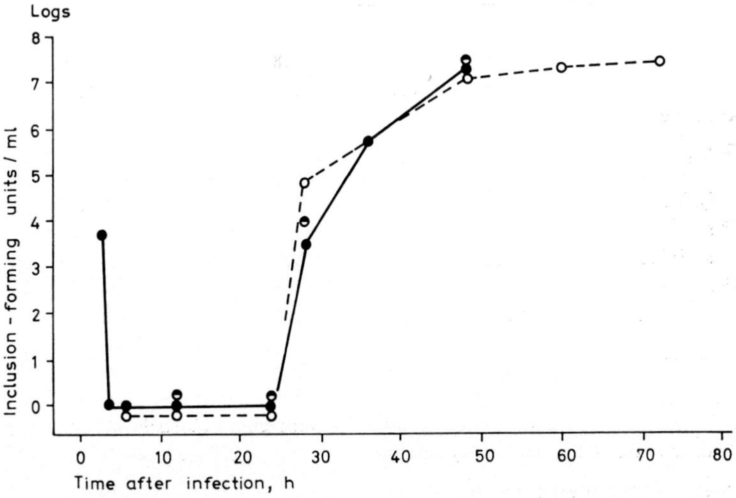

Fig. 3. Three growth curve experiments carried out with the T'ang strain of trachoma in FL cell cultures. ◓ = Curve I; ○ = curve II; ● = curve III. From BERNKOPF and MASHIAH [1962].

into the host cells (phase 1) was due to the initiation of metabolic processes in them. Phase 2 is the period of the development of large inclusions [FURNESS *et al.*, 1962], while phase 3 might correspond to the formation of the e.b. progeny in the inclusion bodies.

B. Factors Affecting C. trachomatis *Development*

1. Nutritional Factors

a) Amino Acids

Due to the intracellular development of the trachoma agent, the amino acids required for its development are supplied by the host cells. Never-

Table IV. Effect of omission of arginine and lysine from medium 12AA on titers of T'ang strain of trachoma, JH strain of LGV, and 6BC strain of psittacosis in FL and HuK cultures

Medium	Titers					
	T'ang		LGV		6 BC	
	FL	HuK	FL	HuK	FL	HuK
LY	100.0	100.0	100.0	100.0	100.0	100.0
12AA	0.5[1]	80.0	0.8	–[2]	83.0	123.0
12AA[3] serine	56.0	85.0	80.0	–	55.0	–
12AA[3] serine – arginine histidine lysine	0.0	0.0	0.0	–	35.7	47.0
12AA[3] serine – arginine	0.2	0.01	0.0	–	–	–
12AA[3] serine – histidine	0.0	0.0	0.0	–	–	–
12AA[3] serine – lysine	0.9	2.9	0.2	–	–	–

6BC = *C. psittaci;* LGV = lymphogranuloma venereum *(C. trachomatis);* T'ang = *C. trachomatis;* HuK = human kidney cell line.

[1] Mean of several experiments.
[2] Not done.
[3] Expressed as percentage of titer in LY medium.
From OSSOWSKI *et al.* [1965].

theless, it was possible to demonstrate [OSSOWSKI *et al.*, 1965] that three strains of *C. trachomatis* (TE 55, Bour and Camal) failed to develop in FL cells grown in Eagle's medium. Addition of serine to this medium resulted in the development of the agents and the formation of up to 71% of the infectious progeny. In this respect, the *C. trachomatis* agents differed from *C. psittaci* which was capable of producing the maximal infectious progeny in infected cells which were incubated in serine-free Eagle's medium. The *C. trachomatis* strains failed to develop when arginine, histidine and lysine were omitted from the medium (table IV). This study demonstrated that *C. trachomatis* agents utilize certain amino acids supplied by the medium in which the cells grow, indicating the inability of the agents to synthesize certain amino acids. These findings might explain in part the obligate parasitism of *C. trachomatis.*

b) Serum

The FL cells were grown in a medium containing 18 amino acids supplemented with 20% human serum [OSSOWSKI *et al.,* 1965]. When the trachoma agent (TE 55)-infected cells were incubated in the same medium but without serum, the development of the infectious progeny was affected [BECKER, 1972a, b]. The factors in the serum which affected trachoma development are not yet known.

2. Temperature of Incubation

FURNESS and FRASER [1962] demonstrated that incubation of trachoma-infected cell cultures at 30 °C resulted in the inhibition of trachoma development. At 30 °C, the synthesis of proteins in the cultured cells is affected, hence the inhibition of trachoma development.

3. The Host Cell

It was shown [OSSOWSKI *et al.,* 1965] that the amino acid requirement of the agent differed according to the host cell. In human kidney cells, *C. trachomatis* agent (TE 55) could produce 80% of its infectivity when the cells were kept in Eagle's medium without serine, but in FL cells no trachoma development took place in the same medium.

Treatment of cultured cells with ionizing irradiation [GORDON and QUAN, 1971] rendered them more susceptible to infection with the trachoma agent.

C. Effects of C. trachomatis *Infection on the Host Cell*

1. Effect on Host Cell Metabolism

Infection of FL cells trachoma agent (TE55) was found not to affect the molecular processes of the host cells [BECKER *et al.*, 1971]. The macromolecular processes of the host cell (DNA, RNA, and protein synthesis) are unaffected in the presence of the trachoma inclusion bodies. As the contribution of *C. trachomatis* to the over-all metabolism of the host cell is small, it was impossible to distinguish trachoma-specific protein synthesis because the infected cells synthesized proteins at a rate similar to that of uninfected cells. Treatment of the cells with the alkaloid emetine made possible the study of the synthesis of trachoma proteins [BECKER and ASHER, 1972b].

2. Induction of Interferon Synthesis

Infection of cultured cells with trachoma e.b. was found [JENKIN and LU, 1966, 1967; MERIGAN and HANNA, 1966; HANNA *et al.*, 1967] to induce interferon synthesis in the treated cells. The response of the infected cells to trachoma e.b., therefore, resembles their reaction to other agents. The interferon induced by the agent in cultured cells had a molecular weight of about 50,000 daltons, hence different from virus-induced interferon [MERIGAN and HANNA, 1966].

D. Morphology of the Developing C. trachomatis *Inclusion Bodies*

1. Correlation between Morphology and Infectivity

FURNESS *et al.* [1962] indicated that a correlation exists between the appearance of DNA-containing particles in the trachoma inclusion body and the appearance of infectious progeny. BERNKOPF *et al.* [1962a] related the developmental cycle of *C. trachomatis* to the morphological events which take place during the morphogenesis of the trachoma agent (TE55). The noninfective phase was characterized by development of inclusion bodies, whereas the infective phase was correlated with the appearance of the elementary bodies [BECKER *et al.*, 1963].

2. Morphology of *C. trachomatis* Inclusions during the Noninfective Phase

The information on the morphology of the developmental cycle of the trachoma agent was derived from studies on fixed preparations of infected cells using electron microscopical techniques. Under these conditions, the morphology of the agent depended on the methods of fixation and sectioning of the infected cells. Early studies [BERNKOPF *et al.*, 1962a; MITSUI *et al.*, 1962b; BECKER *et al.*, 1963; HIGASHI, 1964] on the ultrastructure of trachoma developing particles provided the basic information on the agents and contributed to a marked confusion as a result of inadequate techniques. The difficulties in the interpretations of the developing structures of the agent affected the understanding of the mechanism of trachoma development. Electron microscopy of infected cells at various time periods after infection [BECKER *et al.*, 1963] revealed within the inclusion bodies membrane-bound initial (or secondary) bodies which became larger with time after infection. In these growing structures, membranes gradually appeared which caused the subdivision of the structures into smaller oval bodies. Thus, the initial body was regarded as the developing trachoma structure in which further metabolic processes occurred. The initial body was defined [LITWIN *et al.*, 1961; PAGE, 1973] as the particle within the inclusions prior to the binary fission step. Due to permanganate fixation, the cellular structures were not well preserved but the membranes were noticeable. It was found that the formation of membranes which appeared in the inclusion bodies to make up the initial bodies was inhibited in the presence of penicillin [BERNKOPF *et al.*, 1962b]. Similar difficulties were encountered in the electron microscopical analyses of MITSUI *et al.* [1962b].

With improved fixation techniques (using glutaraldehyde as a fixative) and staining with uranyl acetate and lead citrate, KRAMER and GORDON [1971] obtained a better resolution of the developmental stages of a genital tract trachoma agent. At 12 h post-infection, initial bodies were observed within the inclusion bodies. The initial bodies were heterogeneous in their appearance: some were spherical whereas others were elongated. Evidence for binary fission was seen among the elongated forms. In the presence of penicillin, the initial bodies were retained but further development was arrested. This finding on the effect of penicillin is in agreement with the morphological studies on the TE55 strain [BERNKOPF *et al.*, 1962a] – namely, the development of undifferentiated inclusion bodies.

Using the same procedure of KRAMER and GORDON [1971], the developmental cycle of the *C. trachomatis* agent (TE55) was investigated. Similar findings on the initial bodies and the presence of forms which divide by a mechanism resembling binary fission were described [BECKER, unpublished results] (fig. 4).

3. The Morphology of *C. trachomatis* Inclusion Bodies during the Infectivity-Increase Phase

The appearance of elementary bodies in the inclusion bodies can be correlated with the increase in the infectivity titer. The morphology of the inclusion bodies, at the time infectivity was detected [KRAMER and GORDON, 1971], provided a further demonstration that the initial bodies divided by a mechanism which resembled binary fission. The smaller initial bodies which were present in the inclusions were not uniform in size; most of them were spherical, with a diameter of about 0.8 μm. The outer envelope of the particles was seen as a loosely fitted membrane. Another membrane, most probably the agent's cell membrane, was seen close to the particle's cytoplasm, which contains numerous ribosomes. Later, an electron-dense nucleoid appeared in the particle, and the cell wall was arranged tightly around the particle's membranes. These particles, which are uniform (0.3 μm) in diameter, are the infectious progeny of trachoma e.b. A similar sequence of events was found with the T'ang strain (TE55) during development in FL cells [BECKER, unpublished].

4. Comparison between *C. trachomatis* Inclusions in Cultured Cells and Conjunctival Cells from Trachoma Patients

MITSUI *et al.* [1958] studied the ultrastructure of trachoma inclusions in conjunctival epithelial cells. Electron micrographs revealed the presence of initial and elementary bodies similar to those reported in trachoma-infected cultured cells [KRAMER and GORDON, 1971] (fig. 4).

5. Isolation and Characterization of *C. trachomatis* Initial Bodies

a) Sucrose Gradient Analysis

Electron microscopy of trachoma inclusion bodies (fig. 4C) reveals particles varying in size: large and small bodies which were designated initial

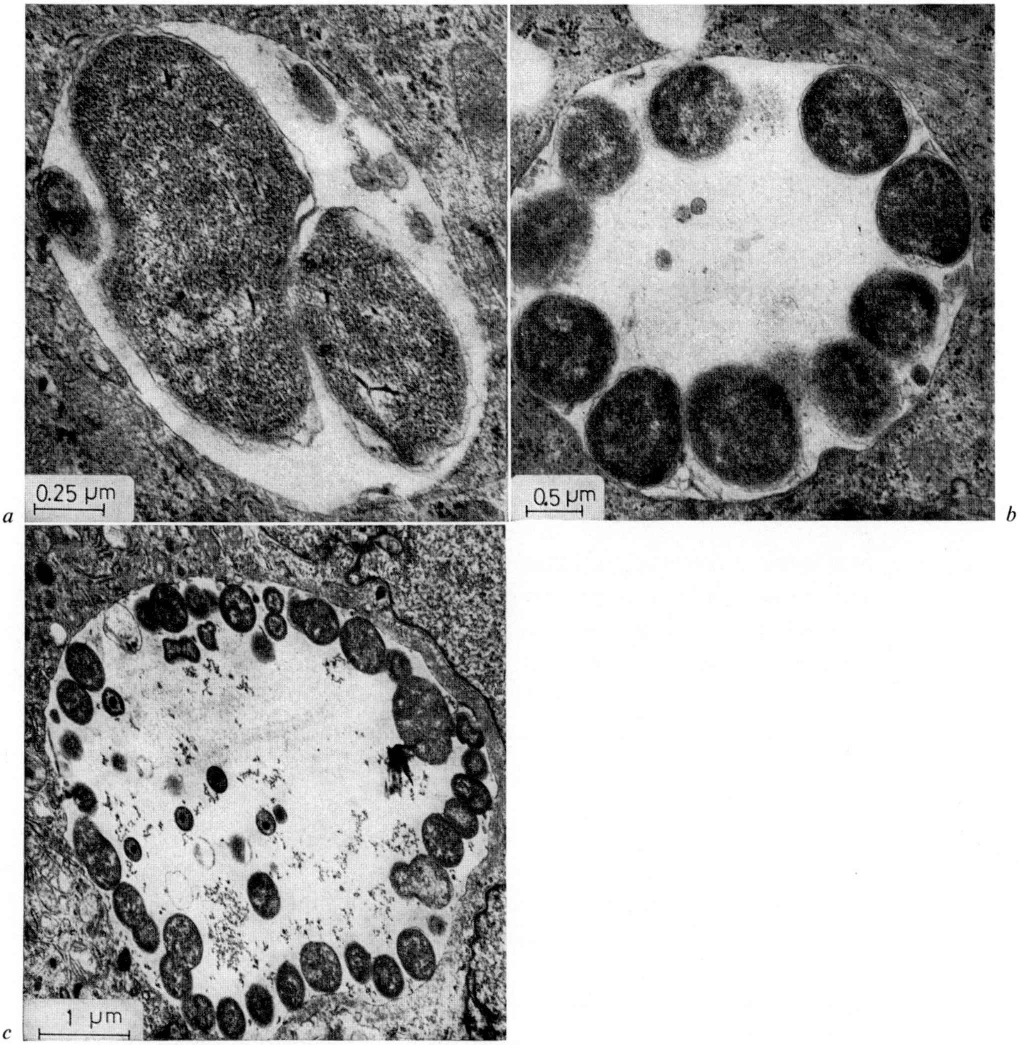

Fig. 4. The developmental cycle of *C. trachomatis* (TE 55 strain) in FL cells. *a* An initial step in the formation of the inclusion body (19 h p.i.). *b* An inclusion body with initial bodies (18 h p.i.). *c* A developed inclusion body with initial bodies, dividing bodies and elementary bodies [BECKER, unpublished].

bodies. Some of these initial bodies can be seen in a binary fission stage. Smaller particles are without a distinct nucleoid while the elementary bodies have a distinct cell wall and a nucleoid. This finding indicated that (a) the developmental cycle is not synchronous and (b) the large initial bodies should differ from the elementary bodies in their hydrodynamic properties when centrifuged in sucrose gradients. Indeed, centrifugation of a homogenate prepared from *C. trachomatis* (TE 55)-infected FL cells in a sucrose gradient revealed that the initial bodies sediment further into the gradient (fig. 5A) than the elementary bodies (fig. 5B). Under these conditions, cell nuclei also band in the gradient together with the initial bodies. Therefore, to purify the initial bodies from cellular components, the nuclei were first centrifuged from the homogenates of the infected cells. One-third of the initial bodies sedimented together with the nuclei. The rest of the initial bodies were retained in the supernatant and were isolated (fig. 5A) by centrifugation in sucrose gradients [Gutter *et al.*, 1973].

b) Characterization of the Initial Bodies

The initial bodies isolated from infected cells after centrifugation in sucrose gradients were stained with phosphotungstic acid and viewed in the electron microscope [Gutter *et al.*, 1973]. Initial bodies which differed in size were isolated from the infected cells. Trachoma agent-specific ribosomal RNA was found to be synthesized in such initial bodies. Similar initial bodies were described by Erlandson and Allen [1964] for the meningopneumonitis agent.

6. Initial Bodies Are Precursors to Elementary Bodies
The Transition of the Initial Bodies to Elementary Bodies

Analysis of mature elementary bodies by centrifugation in a sucrose gradient is presented in figure 5B. Due to the non-synchrony of the *C. trachomatis* developmental cycle, it was essential to develop a technique to synchronize the development of the initial bodies. Studies on the effect of hydroxyurea, an inhibitor of prokaryotic and eukaryotic cellular DNA synthesis [Rosenkranz and Levi, 1965], revealed that treatment of the TE 55 strain-infected FL cells with 5×10^{-4} M hydroxyurea resulted in the inhibition of the formation of elementary bodies. In such cells, the initial bodies accumulated in the inclusion bodies, but they lacked the ability to divide in the absence of DNA synthesis [Rosenkranz *et al.*, 1973]. Homogenates prepared from

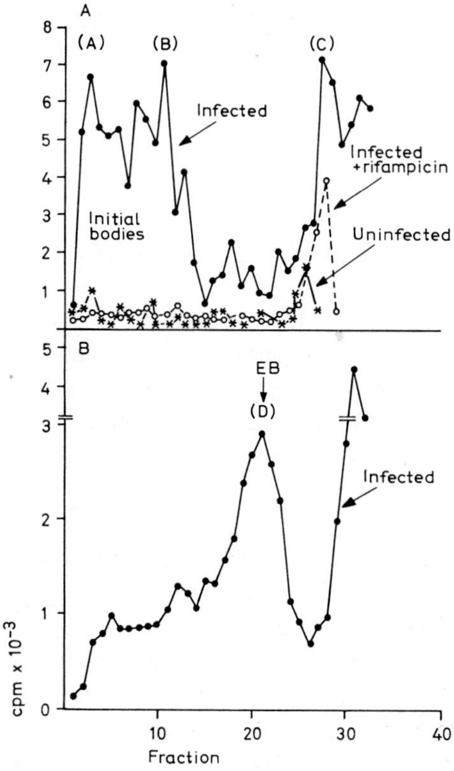

Fig. 5. Isolation of *C. trachomatis* initial bodies and elementary bodies by centrifugation in sucrose gradients. *A* Initial bodies from *C. trachomatis*-infected cells (●). Uninfected cells (○) and rifampicin-treated, infected cells (∗) served as controls. *B* Isolation of elementary bodies (EB) from infected cells. From GUTTER *et al.* [1973].

infected cells treated with hydroxyurea (5×10^{-4} M) were centrifuged in a sucrose gradient and the initial bodies were isolated. To determine the relationship between the initial bodies and the elementary bodies, hydroxyurea-treated *C. trachomatis* (TE 55)-infected cells were labeled with ^{3}H-cytidine. At 48 h after infection, the cells were washed free of the radioisotope and hydroxyurea and were reincubated for an additional period of 12 h. The cells were homogenized and the content of the inclusion bodies was determined by centrifugation in a sucrose gradient. It was found that almost all of the radioactive initial bodies were converted into elementary bodies. This result demonstrated that the initial bodies are the precursors to the elementary bodies.

V. The Composition of Trachoma Elementary Bodies (e.b.)

A. Isolation and Purification of e.b.

Chemical, molecular and antigenic analyses of trachoma e.b. must be carried out on highly purified particles after isolation from the cellular material. The trachoma agent elementary bodies were purified from infected yolk sacs or from infected cultured cells by several techniques, of which zonal centrifugation in sucrose gradients became one of the methods of choice.

1. Purification of e.b. from Infected Yolk Sacs

a) Sucrose Gradient Centrifugation

WANG *et al.* [1967b] and WANG and GRAYSTON [1967b] isolated e.b. from *C. trachomatis*-infected yolk sac material by centrifugation of the latter in continuous sucrose gradients (0–40% sucrose) containing 1.0 M KCl. The gradients were centrifuged at 1,500 *g* for 2 h and the dense zones, which contained e.b., were obtained. Further purification of e.b. was attained, although not all the yolk material was removed, by ZAKAY-RONES *et al.* [1969] using zonal rotors for centrifugation of the infected yolk sac material in sucrose gradients.

b) DEAE-Sephadex Column Chromatography [WANG and GRAYSTON, 1967a, b]

A suspension of infected yolk sac material, partially purified by several cycles of differential centrifugation, was put on a DEAE-sephadex column and eluted with 0.35–0.4 M NaCl solution containing sucrose (0.4 M) and phosphate buffer. The eluate was subjected to one cycle of differential centrifugation in phosphate-buffered saline. The elementary bodies thus obtained were infectious.

c) Genetron Treatment

WANG and GRAYSTON [1967b] purified a suspension of elementary bodies from yolk sac material by mixing in a blender with Genetron 113 or Genesolv-D (trifluorotrichloroethane). After centrifugation at 500 *g* for 10 min, the top aqueous layer was collected and the procedure was repeated. Infectivity was lost by genetron treatment.

2. Isolation of e. b. from Infected Cultured Cells

The isolation of e. b. from infected cultured cells was achieved by the sucrose gradient technique. The initial purification step was to centrifuge the homogenate of infected cells into a sucrose gradient prepared on top of a sucrose cushion. The e. b. which banded on top of the sucrose cushion were removed, diluted and recentrifuged in a second sucrose gradient. The opalescent band of particles was removed for further studies. The infectivity of the e. b. was retained [Sarov and Becker, 1968].

Zonal centrifugation in sucrose gradients was developed as a technique for the isolation of *C. trachomatis* e. b. from infected yolk sac material or cultured cells. Large quantities of e. b. can be obtained with the aid of zonal rotors, which might enhance the preparation of antitrachoma vaccines. However, purified preparations still contain yolk sac material which, most probably, adhered to the surface of the e. b. The e. b. purified by the sucrose gradient technique retained their infectivity and provided a good source of e. b. for further research.

B. The Chemical Composition of Trachoma e. b.

The e. b. of *C. trachomatis* are capable of development in the cytoplasm of the host cells. Thus, they must contain the genetic apparatus which controls their growth and development. Chemical analyses of the e. b. may, therefore, shed light on the properties of the agent and the molecular mechanisms involved in the initiation and synthesis of the agent's progeny.

1. The DNA Genome

a) The Molecular Weight of the DNA Genome

DNA molecules were isolated from the TE55 strain of *C. trachomatis* by a procedure which minimized shearing and yielded high molecular weight circular DNA molecules [SAROV and BECKER, 1969]. The molecular weight of trachoma DNA was found to be 660 × 10^6 daltons (11 × 10^5 nucleotide pairs) determined both by electron microscopy and sedimentation in sucrose gradients. A lower value (6 × 10^5 nucleotide pairs) was reported by KINGSBURY [1969] for the DNA of the MRC-1/G strain of *C. trachomatis*. However, while the measurements of trachoma DNA by SAROV and BECKER [1969] were based on the size of the DNA as measured from the electron micrographs of the DNA preparations, KINGSBURY's determination was based on a less accurate method, the reassociation between single-stranded DNA fragments. KINGSBURY [1969] had also demonstrated that the *C. psittaci* DNA genome contains 8.5 × 10^5 nucleotide pairs (473 × 10^6 daltons molecular weight), while TAMURA [1964a, b] reported that the meningopneumonitis agent DNA has a molecular weight of 9.5 × 10^8 daltons. A comparison between the genome size of various microorganisms and *C. trachomatis* was presented by WEISS [1971].

The molecular weight of trachoma DNA [SAROV and BECKER, 1969] is (a) about 4 times larger than vaccinia virus DNA (150 × 10^6 daltons) [BECKER and SAROV, 1968], (b) larger than the DNA genome of *Mycoplasma hominis* (8.5 × 10^5 nucleotide base pairs) [BODE and MOROWITZ, 1967], and (c) one-fourth of *E. coli* DNA [CAIRNS, 1963]. Thus, the genetic information of *C. trachomatis* is organized in a circular DNA molecule present in the e.b. From the molecular size of the DNA, it is possible to conclude that it contains genetic information for several hundred different proteins, which are still to be characterized. The complete analysis of the developmental cycle might provide us with a clue to the evolution of *C. trachomatis* and its obligate parasitism.

b) Properties of C. trachomatis *DNA*

The guanosine + cytosine (G + C) content of DNA provides an indication regarding the composition of the DNA genome. It was found [WEISS *et al.*, 1970] that the G + C content in *C. trachomatis* DNA was 42.5%, while *C. psittaci* DNA contained 39.5% G + C. The differences in base composition between the two species were reflected also in the results of the DNA reassociation experiments [WEISS *et al.*, 1970]. Analysis of the *C. trachomatis* (TE55 strain) DNA revealed that the primary shearing products were fragments of about one-third of the genome [SAROV and BECKER, 1969]. It was suggested that the trachoma DNA might have cross-linkages in the DNA, which were sensitive to shearing. The biological significance of this property of the DNA is not yet known.

2. RNA in the e. b.

a) Ribosomal Subunits

Treatment of purified *C. trachomatis* (TE 55 strain) e. b., labeled with ^{3}H-cytidine in the agent's nucleic acids, with the detergent sodium deoxycholate released the content of the particles. Analysis by centrifugation in sucrose gradients revealed the presence of labeled 30S and 52S ribosomal subunits. No ribosomes were detected in the e. b. by this procedure [SAROV and BECKER, 1968]. Ribosomal subunits with sedimentation constants of 50S and 30S were also isolated from the psittacosis agent [TAMURA, 1967]. The reason for the presence of 30S and 52S ribosomal subunits in the TE 55 e. b. is not known. It is tempting to suggest that the ribosomal subunits will associate to form ribosomes only after the initiation of mRNA synthesis during the development of the e. b. in the infected host cell.

b) Ribosomal RNA

Analysis of the RNA molecules extracted from TE 55 e. b., labeled with ^{3}H-cytidine, by sedimentation in sucrose gradients [SAROV and BECKER, 1968] or by electrophoresis in acrylamide gels [BECKER *et al.*, 1971; GUTTER and BECKER, 1972] revealed RNA species with sedimentation constants of 23S (1.1×10^6 daltons molecular weight) and 16S (0.55×10^6 daltons molecular weight), which resembled the ribosomal RNA species of *C. psittaci* [TAMURA and IWANAGA, 1965] and *E. coli.* The 52S ribosomal subunits contained the 23S RNA molecules while the 30S contained the 16S RNA species [SAROV and BECKER, 1968].

The acrylamide gel electropherograms revealed that 5S RNA molecules, which are associated with the ribosomes, were also present in the e. b. The function of this RNA species is not yet known.

c) Transfer RNA

Electropherograms of the RNA species extracted from trachoma (TE 55) e. b. revealed the presence of 4S RNA molecules in the e. b. [GUTTER and BECKER, 1972]. The amino acid acceptor activities of these 4S RNA molecules have not yet been studied.

d) Messenger RNA

It is not yet known if the e. b. of *C. trachomatis* contain mRNA species or if mRNA molecules are transcribed by the endogenous DNA-dependent RNA polymerase after entry of the e. b. into the host cells. In the electropherograms of RNA from e. b., RNA species which differed from the ribosomal RNA, 5S and transfer RNA species were seen [GUTTER and BECKER, 1972] but their nature has not yet been studied.

3. Proteins in e. b.

The presence of ribosomal subunits in *C. trachomatis* e. b. indicated that they might contain a large number of ribosomal proteins as well as other structural proteins. To characterize the proteins, purified e. b. were prepared from FL cells infected with *C. trachomatis* (TE55 strain) grown in the absence or the presence of ^{14}C-amino acids. The purified suspensions of e. b. were treated with a solution of sodium dodecyl sulfate (SDS), urea and 2-mercaptoethanol and analyzed by electrophoresis in acrylamide gels [MAIZEL, 1966]. The electropherograms of the unlabeled e. b. revealed, after staining with Coomassie blue, 20 protein bands, which correspond to 38 bands observed in the electropherograms of radioactively labeled e. b. proteins [BECKER *et al.*, 1971]. It was possible to assume that only part of the e. b. proteins were revealed in these analyses. The nature and function of these and other proteins are not yet known.

4. Lipids in the e. b.

JENKIN [1967] analyzed the lipid composition of *C. trachomatis* e. b. (TW-3 strain) which were adapted to growth in HeLa cells [JENKIN, 1966]. It was found that the trachoma e. b. contained the same phospholipids as the HeLa cells, possibly because the e. b. were purified by differential centrifugation only, and not by banding in sucrose gradients to reduce the contamination with host cell components. It was not possible to compare the lipid composition of trachoma e. b. to that of psittacosis agent e. b. because the two organisms were grown in different hosts, and the contamination with host cell lipids might have affected the analyses. Recently, it was found [BECKER, unpublished] that when *C. trachomatis* (TE55 strain) was grown in FL cells in the presence of ^{3}H-choline in the medium, the purified e. b. (after banding in sucrose gradients) contained choline-labeled lipids. The nature of these lipids has not yet been studied.

5. Cell Membranes and Cell Walls in Trachoma e. b.

Electron microscopy of *C. trachomatis* e. b. revealed the presence of a distinct cell wall around the e. b., as well as a distinct cell membrane. The chemical composition of the cell wall and the cell membrane has not yet been established.

Studies on *C. psittaci* [meningopneumonitis agent; MOULDER 1962, 1966] demonstrated that (a) muramic acid, a constituent of the bacterial cell wall mucopeptide, has been identified in psittacosis agents [PERKINS and ALLISON, 1963]; (b) lysine was present in meningopneumonitis cell wall while diaminopimelic acid was absent [MOULDER, 1966]; and (c) the cell walls contain peptidoglycans [TRIBBY, 1970]. However, it has not yet been determined whether the *C. trachomatis* e. b. cell wall composition resembles that of *C. psittaci.*

C. Antigenic Composition of Trachoma e. b.

1. Antigens

The e. b. of *C. trachomatis* strains (G-17, TW-5) and mouse pneumonitis agent *(C. psittaci)* were used for the preparation of various antigenic fractions for immunization of rabbits [KUO *et al.*, 1971a]. Using the double immunodiffusion test, up to seven distinct antigenic components were recognized in *C. trachomatis* as well as in *C. psittaci.* Three antigens were heat-stable group-specific antigens; two of these were solubilized by deoxycholate and the third one was a cell wall antigen [KUO *et al.*, 1971a]. A similar number of antigens were found in *C. trachomatis* by KATZENELSON and BERNKOPF [1967]. BARRON and COLLINS [1967] and COLLINS and BARRON [1970] extracted the group-specific antigen by sodium deoxycholate treatment of *C. trachomatis* e. b. and demonstrated its antigenicity by gel diffusion. Treatment of e. b. with neuraminidase enhanced the antigenic properties [PETERS, 1967].

2. Chemical Composition of the Group-Specific Antigen

DHIR *et al.* [1972] extracted an acidic polysaccharide of a large molecular weight from *C. psittaci* (psittacosis agent) and *C. trachomatis* (lymphogranuloma venereum and trachoma agents). The isolated compound, which retained its antigenicity, was defined as 2-keto-3-deoxyoctanoic acid. The antigenicity of the compound was destroyed by periodate and mild acid hydrolysis.

3. Hemagglutinin

Homogenization of *C. trachomatis* e.b. (TE 55 and Bour strains) by sonic treatment revealed a hemagglutinin which agglutinated at 37 °C (but not at 4 °C) chicken erythrocytes sensitive to the psittacosis agent and vaccinia virus hemagglutinins. The hemagglutinin was inactivated by 0.1 % $MgSO_4$, chloroform or trypsin, and by homologous antibodies as well as antipsittacosis antibodies. The hemagglutinin might be the group-specific antigen [ZAKAY-RONES *et al.*, 1968] similar to that of the psittacosis agent [BARRON *et al.*, 1965].

4. Toxin

A toxic material was obtained from *C. trachomatis*-infected cells [reviewed by BERNKOPF, 1962]. The toxin [MITSUI *et al.*, 1962a] was antigenically different in different strains. Immunization of mice against trachoma resulted in the synthesis of specific antibodies which neutralized the toxin. This phenomenon was utilized in the mouse toxicity prevention test (MTPT) [TAVERNE *et al.*, 1964; WANG and GRAYSTON, 1967a, b].

D. Enzymatic Activities in Trachoma e.b.

The e.b. of *C. trachomatis* are the infectious entity of the agent, capable of adsorption to and infection of sensitive eukaryotic cells. The e.b. develop into a larger, active form after entry into the infected host cell; they are capable of initiating certain metabolic processes after entry into the cell, probably prior to synthesis of new proteins. The presence of enzymes in the e.b. might be associated with the initiation of its development in the eukaryotic cell.

1. DNA-Dependent RNA Polymerase

The demonstration by BECKER and ZAKAY-RONES [1969] that rifampicin, a potent inhibitor of prokaryotic DNA-dependent RNA polymerase [WEHRLI

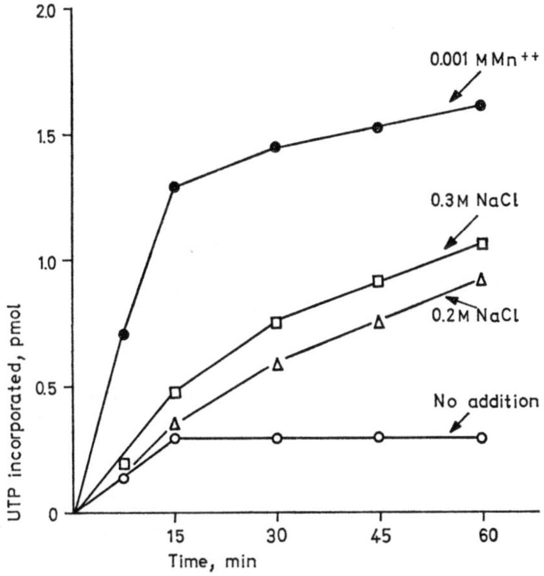

Fig. 6. Effect of Mn^{++} and NaCl on the kinetics of RNA synthesis by trachoma elementary bodies. The reaction mixture (about 2.5×10^7 elementary bodies), containing 0.004 M Mg^{++}, Tris-buffer and the nucleoside triphosphates ('no addition' = ○), and either Mn^{++} (●) or NaCl (0.2 M = △; 0.3 M = □), was incubated at 36 °C for various periods. Samples were removed at different times. Each point represents the average of three determinations. From SAROV and BECKER [1971a].

and STAEHELIN, 1969], inhibited trachoma agent development suggested that the trachoma agent might contain such an enzyme. To study this enzymatic activity, highly purified e. b. preparations (TE 55 strain) were treated with a detergent (sodium deoxycholate) and 2-mercaptoethanol, and were incubated at 37 °C in the presence of ATP, GTP, CTP, ^{3}H-UTP, Mg^{++} and Mn^{++} in Tris–HCl buffer, pH 7.7. Under these conditions, RNA molecules with a sedimentation coefficient of 11–17S were synthesized. Addition of 0.2 M NaCl, instead of Mn^{++}, to the reaction mixture resulted in the prolonged synthesis of elongated (24S) RNA molecules (fig. 6) [SAROV and BECKER, 1971a, b]. Treatment of purified e. b. with 2-mercaptoethanol (without the detergent) caused the release of RNA polymerase molecules from the e. b. These enzyme molecules were completely inhibited by rifampicin [BECKER *et al.*, 1971].

2. Polynucleotide Phosphorylase

In addition to the DNA-dependent RNA polymerase released from 2-mercaptoethanol-treated trachoma e.b. [SAROV and BECKER, 1971b], another enzymatic activity was demonstrable. This enzyme was capable of polymerizing ^{3}H-UTP in the absence of GTP, CTP and ATP. The molecules of this enzyme had a faster sedimentation rate in the sucrose gradient as compared to the RNA polymerase. The nature and role of this enzyme in the development of the e.b. is not yet known [SAROV and BECKER, 1971b].

3. Enzymes for Glucose Metabolism

A number of enzymatic activities were found in *C. trachomatis* and *C. psittaci* elementary bodies isolated from infected yolk sacs [reviewed by MOULDER, 1966, and WEISS, 1971]. It was shown [WEISS, 1967a, b] that the trachoma agent e.b. (TW-55) catabolized glutamate. Glucose was metabolized only after it was converted to glucose-6-phosphate by added hexokinase and adenosine triphosphate [WEISS *et al.*, 1970]. Glucose-6-phosphate was metabolized by the pentose and the glycolytic pathways. The two enzymes involved, which were present in purified e.b. (glucose-6-phosphate and 6-phosphogluconate dehydrogenases), were stimulated by the addition of the cofactor nicotinamide adenine dinucleotide phosphate (NADP). Chlamydiae did not reoxidize NADP [WEISS, 1967a, b]. Preparations of *C. trachomatis* agents resembled *C. psittaci* agents in their ability to metabolize glucose [WEISS *et al.*, 1964].

4. Transaminase Activity

Trachoma e.b. (prepared from infected yolk sacs) were shown to produce CO_2 from the C_1 positions of pyruvate and glutamate but not from other carbon atoms. The reaction of trachoma with glutamate was greatly enhanced by added NADP [WEISS, 1967b].

VI. Molecular Aspects of the Developmental Cycle of *C. trachomatis*

A. Initiation of e.b. Development after Infection of Eukaryotic Cells

1. Initiation of RNA Synthesis in the e.b.

Acridine orange staining of the elementary bodies of *C. trachomatis* and *C. psittaci* revealed, on observation in the UV microscope, a green fluorescence [POLLARD *et al.*, 1960b; POLLARD and TANAMI, 1962] suggesting the presence of DNA molecules in the e.b. POLLARD and TANAMI [1962], COLLIER [1962] and BERNKOPF *et al.* [1962a] reported that the staining reaction changed from green to red, suggesting an active synthesis of RNA. COLLIER [1962] reported that as early as 3 h after adsorption to the cells the e.b. of inclusion blennorrhea demonstrated a red fluorescence (RNA synthesis). These studies suggested that one of the early processes which occurred in the e.b. after entry into the host cell cytoplasm was the synthesis of RNA molecules. The nature of the newly synthesized RNA molecules and the enzyme responsible for RNA transcription were revealed 9 years later.

2. Activation of the e.b.-Associated DNA-Dependent RNA Polymerase

The DNA-dependent RNA polymerase molecules which were shown to exist in the e.b. were activated after entry of the e.b. into the host cell cytoplasm. This was demonstrated by the inhibitory effect of rifampicin on the development of the e.b. [BECKER and ZAKAY-RONES, 1969]. It was assumed [BECKER, 1972a, b] that the RNA polymerase molecules were activated in the e.b. by the availability of the four nucleoside triphosphates which were obtained from the cytoplasm.

3. The Role of Host Cell Mitochondria in e.b. Development

To test if the trachoma e.b. needed the host cell for the supply of the nucleoside triphosphates necessary for RNA synthesis, the effect of ethidium bromide on the development of trachoma e. b. was studied [BECKER and ASHER, 1972a]. It was found that the trachoma agent failed to develop in eukaryotic cells pretreated with the drug. These results are taken to indicate that mitochondrial functions are essential for trachoma development. Further studies [BECKER, unpublished] also demonstrated that treatment of purified trachoma e. b. with ethidium bromide resulted in the inhibition of e. b. development, indicating that ethidium bromide molecules intercalated into the trachoma DNA and prevented the transcription of the e. b. DNA genomes.

4. Initiation of Protein Synthesis in the e. b.

Subsequent to RNA synthesis in the e. b., which occurs 6 h after entry into the host cell cytoplasm, the synthesis of peptides begins. Addition to *C. trachomatis* (TE 55)-infected cells of the antibiotic pactamycin (an inhibitor of peptide chain initiation) at a concentration of 0.01 μg/ml completely inhibited the development of the agent [BECKER, unpublished].

B. RNA Synthesis during the Trachoma Developmental Cycle

1. Cytoplasmic Site of RNA Synthesis in the *C. trachomatis*-Infected Cell

Labeling of TE 55-infected cells with ^{3}H-uridine resulted in the incorporation of the isotope into RNA molecules synthesized in the trachoma inclusion bodies. Radioautography of FL cells infected with *C. trachomatis* and labeled with ^{3}H-uridine during the initial 24 h after infection revealed that grains were localized on the inclusion bodies in the cytoplasm and in the nucleoli in the host cell nuclei [BERNKOPF *et al.*, 1962a]. This finding demonstrated that RNA synthesis in the inclusion bodies was not dependent on host cell nucleolar RNA synthesis.

2. Rate of *C. trachomatis* RNA Synthesis

The rate of RNA synthesis in the developing trachoma (TE 55) agent was studied by GUTTER and BECKER [1972] by labeling the infected cells with ^{3}H-cytidine for 20-min-periods at different time intervals after infection.

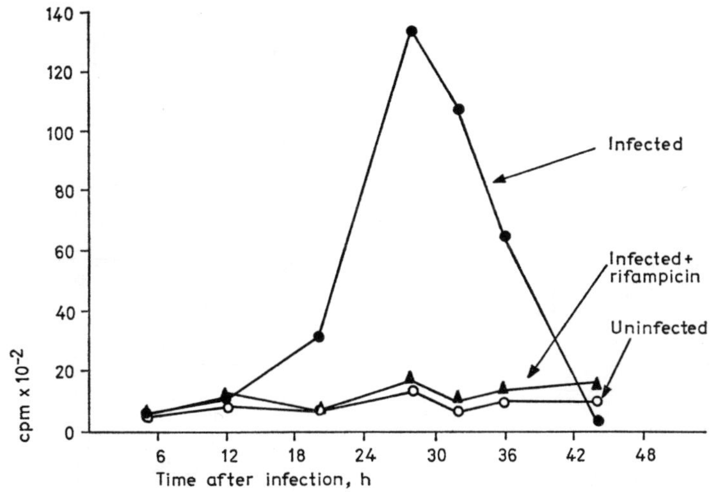

Fig. 7. Rate of RNA synthesis in *C. trachomatis* (TE55)-infected FL cells (●). Uninfected cells (○) and rifampicin-treated, infected cells (▲) served as controls [GUTTER, unpublished].

It was found that (a) trachoma agent RNA synthesis was not distinguishable from that of the host cell during the initial 12 h after infection, (b) from 12 to 30 h a gradual increase in the rate of RNA synthesis took place and (c) the rate of RNA synthesis sharply declined thereafter (fig. 7). RNA synthesis was inhibited by rifampicin.

3. Synthesis of Precursors to Ribosomal RNA

Analysis of the RNA species synthesized in the initial bodies of *C. trachomatis* (TE55) agent by electrophoresis in acrylamide gels revealed a new species of RNA (designated 17.2S) in addition to the trachoma-specific 16S RNA. This RNA species, which resembles the precursor to 16S RNA species reported in bacteria, is the precursor to the trachoma 16S RNA. Another ribosomal RNA species which was synthesized by the trachoma agent consisted of 23S RNA molecules. No precursor molecules to the 23S RNA species were found [GUTTER and BECKER, 1972]. This finding emphasizes the prokaryotic nature of *C. trachomatis*.

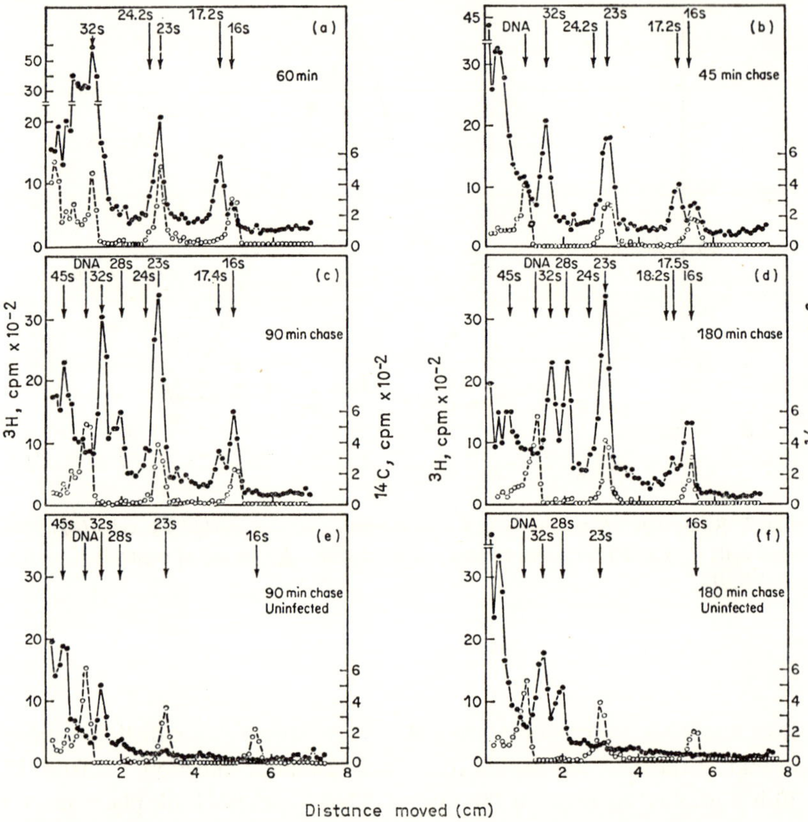

Fig. 8. Maturation of trachoma RNA. Trachoma-infected cells at 24 h post-infection were treated for 2 h with emetine and then labeled with (^{3}H)-cytidine for 60 min (a). A sample of cells was washed with buffer to remove the isotope and reincubated in fresh medium containing unlabeled cytidine (chase experiment). The cells were incubated for 45 min (b), 90 min (c) and 180 min (d) and were then sampled for analysis. Uninfected cells were also labeled for 60 min and incubated for 90 min (e) and 180 min (f) in the absence of the isotope. The cells were dissolved with sodium dodecyl sulphate and analyzed on 3% polyacrylamide gels (●). Trachoma e.b. ribosomal RNA, labeled with (^{14}C)-uridine (○) served as internal marker. From GUTTER and BECKER [1972].

4. Maturation of Trachoma Ribosomal RNA

The nature of the 17.2S trachoma RNA species was studied in emetine-treated, infected cells; the alkaloid drug emetine inhibits the synthesis of host cell RNA without affecting trachoma development [BECKER and ASHER, 1972b]. Analysis of the labeled trachoma RNA molecules after removal of the radioactive precursor (^{3}H-cytidine) resulted in the processing of the 17.2S molecules, which yielded 16S RNA species. During this process, the amount of radioactivity in the 23S trachoma rRNA gradually increased, although no larger radioactive RNA species were synthesized. This result also suggested that a precursor to trachoma 23S exists, although not yet revealed. The processing of the precursor molecules depended on protein synthesis and was inhibited in the presence of inhibitors of protein synthesis [GUTTER and BECKER, 1972] (fig. 8).

The finding that the 16S ribosomal RNA of *C. trachomatis* (TE55 strain) is formed after the cleavage of 17.2S RNA precursor molecules reveals its resemblance to prokaryotic cells. A similar situation was found to exist in *E. coli* [ADESNIK and LEVINTHAL, 1969]: the 23S ribosomal RNA molecules and the 16S ribosomal RNA molecules are formed after the cleavage of 24S and 17.2S precursor molecules, respectively. The slow processing of the *C. trachomatis* 17.2S to 16S (about 2 h are needed for the conversion of 17.2S to 16S rRNA species, while only several minutes are required in *E. coli*) might give an explanation for the slow developmental cycle of the agent [GUTTER and BECKER, 1972].

5. Synthesis of Trachoma 5S and 4S RNA Species

In addition to the 16S, 17.2S and 23S ribosomal RNA species, the developing *C. trachomatis* agent (TE55 strain) also synthesizes 5S and 4S RNA species. This finding might indicate that the t-RNA species present in the developing trachoma structures are coded by the agent, but it is not yet known if t-RNA species to all amino acids are synthesized by the agent.

6. RNA Synthesis in the Initial (Secondary) Bodies

Analysis by acrylamide gel electrophoresis of RNA species synthesized in *C. trachomatis* (TE55)-infected cells revealed the synthesis of 23S and 17.2S RNA species. The latter serves as a precursor to 16S ribosomal RNA. The synthesis of these RNA species was inhibited by rifampicin, indicating

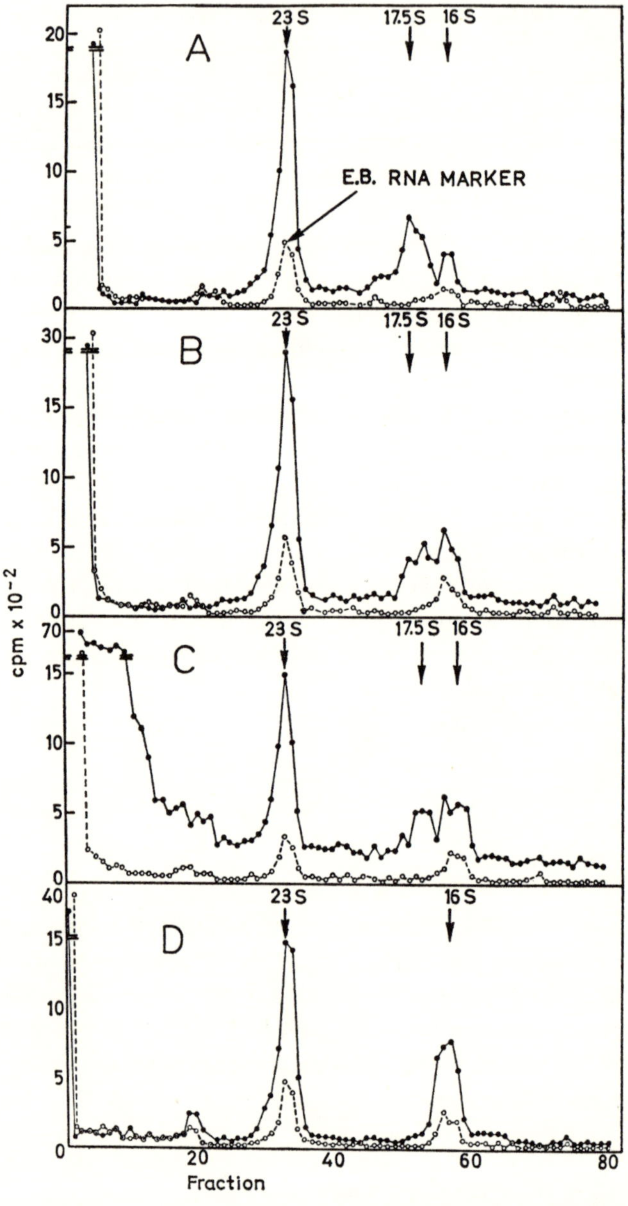

Fig. 9. Acrylamide gel analyses of RNA species synthesized in the initial bodies. A, B, C, and D are the analyses of the RNA species in samples from the pooled bands marked (A), (B), (C), and (D) in the sucrose density gradients presented in figure 5A and B. The RNA species present in each sample were determined by electrophoresis in acrylamide gels. From GUTTER *et al.* [1973].

their prokaryotic nature. Isolation of the initial bodies by centrifugation in a sucrose gradient made possible the determination of the site of RNA synthesis in the trachoma inclusion bodies. It was found [GUTTER *et al.*, 1973] that the different RNA species of the trachoma agent are synthesized in the initial bodies (fig. 9A, B, C). The elementary bodies contain only the mature 23S and the 16S ribosomal RNA species (fig. 90).

7. DNA-Dependent RNA Polymerase in the Purified Initial Bodies

The purified initial bodies were incubated with dithiothreitol and the four nucleoside triphosphates to assay for an RNA-synthesizing activity. It was found that RNA was synthesized *in vitro*, and this process was inhibited by actinomycin D and rifampicin [BECKER and ASHER, to be published]. These results demonstrated that the initial bodies contain the DNA genomes of *C. trachomatis,* which are transcribed by a specific prokaryotic DNA-dependent RNA polymerase.

C. DNA Synthesis

1. Time Course of DNA Synthesis

Determination of DNA synthesis in the developing inclusion bodies of the TE55 agent with the aid of the Feulgen technique revealed DNA synthesis later than 24 h after infection. Similar findings were obtained by determining DNA content in infected cells [BECKER *et al.*, 1962]. Recent studies [BECKER *et al.*, 1971] demonstrated that the rate of DNA synthesis markedly increased during the period 24–36 h after infection and sharply declined thereafter. In this study, the rate of DNA synthesis was studied by determining the amount of alkali-resistant ^{3}H-cytidine-labeled nucleic acids.

2. Site of DNA Synthesis

Analysis of nascent DNA molecules present in the trachoma agent (TE55) was carried out by the separation of the secondary bodies from the e.b. after labeling with ^{3}H-cytidine. It was found [ROSENKRANZ *et al.*, 1973] that the secondary bodies do not contain labeled DNA molecules. Only the particles present in the e.b. band in the sucrose gradient contain labeled DNA molecules. It is assumed that DNA synthesis is coupled with the transformation of the trachoma initial bodies to elementary bodies. This result assumes that trachoma DNA is synthesized in conjunction with the synthesis of membranes, as reported for prokaryotic cells. However, direct information regarding the maturation of trachoma secondary bodies into e.b. is still lacking.

3. DNA Synthesis and Morphogenesis

The development of trachoma agent elementary bodies in the infected cells was found to be dependent on the initiation of RNA synthesis in the infecting particles [BECKER, 1972a, b]. The requirement for DNA synthesis during the initial period of development of elementary bodies was revealed with the aid of hydroxyurea. Treatment of *C. trachomatis*-infected (TE55) cells with 5×10^{-2} M hydroxyurea completely inhibited the development of the e.b. in the infected cells [ROSENKRANZ *et al.*, 1973]. This result was taken to indicate that the development of trachoma e.b. is coupled with the replication of the agent's DNA genome. The synthesis of DNA is required throughout the developmental cycle of the agent. The inhibitory effect of 5×10^{-4} M hydroxyurea on the formation of e.b. suggested that the duplication of the agent's DNA genome is indeed required for the transformation of the initial bodies into e.b. No information is available as yet regarding the enzymatic processes involved in the synthesis of trachoma DNA and the site of DNA duplication in the initial bodies. Preliminary studies [BECKER, unpublished data] demonstrated the presence of a DNA-dependent DNA polymerase activity in the TE55 initial bodies.

D. Protein Synthesis

1. Time Course of *C. trachomatis* Protein Synthesis

The synthesis of *C. trachomatis* proteins could not be detected in the infected cells because the trachoma agent proteins comprised less than 10% of the cellular proteins. It was essential to devise ways to inhibit the cellular protein synthesis without affecting the parasite. Treatment of *C. trachomatis*-infected cells with cycloheximide partially reduced cellular protein synthesis, but not enough to detect the trachoma-specific processes [BECKER *et al.*,

1971]. Further studies [BECKER and ASHER, 1972b] demonstrated that the alkaloid emetine (at 50 μg/ml) almost completely inhibited host cell protein synthesis and made possible the study of trachoma-specific protein synthesis. Pulse labeling of emetine-treated infected cells demonstrated that during the initial 18 h after infection it was not possible to distinguish between trachoma and host protein synthesis. The rate of trachoma protein synthesis sharply increased during the period from 20 to 42 h after infection. Later on, the rate of protein synthesis markedly declined. The synthesis of proteins was found to stop at 48 h p.i. when the formation of e.b. was completed [BECKER and ASHER, 1972b]. Similar results were obtained when cellular protein synthesis was inhibited by anisomycin [BECKER, unpublished].

2. Characterization of Trachoma Proteins Synthesized in Infected Cells

To characterize trachoma proteins synthesized during the developmental cycle, the infected cells were labeled for 6-hour periods at different stages of the agent's growth cycle. After labeling, the radioactive precursor was removed from the medium and the infected cells were incubated in fresh medium. The progeny of e.b. was obtained at 48 h after infection and the proteins, which were incorporated into the e.b., were analyzed by electrophoresis in acrylamide gels. It was found [BECKER *et al.*, 1971] that different species of proteins were synthesized at different phases of the developmental cycle. Analysis of the trachoma proteins synthesized in emetine-treated trachoma-infected cells, in which cellular protein synthesis was markedly inhibited, also revealed the various species of *C. trachomatis*-specific proteins. The nature of these proteins and their function are still to be studied.

E. Glycogen Synthesis

1. Demonstration of Glycogen in the Inclusions of *C. trachomatis*

RICE [1935] demonstrated that the inclusion bodies of *C. trachomatis* contained polysaccharide molecules which were stained by iodine (probably glycogen). The synthesis of glycogen in the inclusion bodies was a feature characteristic of the agents which belonged to *C. trachomatis* [subgroup A of GORDON and QUAN, 1965a, b] and served to differentiate the latter from the agents of *C. psittaci* (subgroup B).

2. Relationship between Glycogen Synthesis and the *C. trachomatis* Growth Cycle

BERNKOPF *et al.* [1962a] studied the time course of the appearance of carbohydrate (presumably glycogen) in the inclusion bodies of the TE55 agent grown in FL cells. It was found that the number of inclusions which were stained with iodine increased sharply during a 10-hour period, starting at 20 h after infection. The inclusion bodies gradually became negative to iodine staining, indicating that the carbohydrate was degraded after synthesis. An indication that carbohydrate synthesis was dependent on the morphogenesis of the agent was obtained from the effect of penicillin. The synthesis of the carbohydrate was prevented in inclusions in which the formation of initial (secondary) bodies was prevented by penicillin treatment.

A direct analysis of glycogen in the inclusion bodies of *C. trachomatis* – trachoma and lymphogranuloma venereum (LGV) agents – was reported by FAN and JENKIN [1970], JENKIN and FAN [1971] and EVANS [1972]. Glycogen accumulated during the developmental cycle of the trachoma agent (TW-3) in infected HeLa cells, but not in psittacosis agent-infected cells. The carbohydrate molecules were labeled with ^{14}C-glucose, extracted from the infected cells, and the radioactivity in the carbohydrate was determined. It was found that the same low level of carbohydrate synthesis occurred in uninfected cells and in cells infected with *C. psittaci* (meningopneumonitis agent). In HeLa cells infected with *C. trachomatis* (TW-3 strain) an increased rate of glycogen synthesis took place during a 24-hour period starting at 48 h after infection. Similarly, in LGV agent-infected cells, a marked increase in carbohydrate synthesis also occurred during the period 24–48 h after infection. The polysaccharide proved to contain maltose and glucose with an average chain length of 11 units [COLLIER, 1973].

3. Effect of Inhibitors on Glycogen Biosynthesis

a) Effect of Penicillin

Addition of penicillin to *C. trachomatis* (TE55)-infected FL cells resulted in a marked inhibition of carbohydrate synthesis as measured by determining the number of inclusion bodies which stained with lugol [BERNKOPF *et al.*, 1962a]. The number of carbohydrate-positive inclusion bodies increased slightly, starting at 30 h after infection.

b) Effect of Fluorouracil on Glycogen Synthesis and Degradation

Treatment of *C. trachomatis* (TE55)-infected FL cells with 1 μg/ml 5-fluorouracil (5FU) resulted in a marked inhibitory effect on the development of trachoma inclusions. However, 80% of the inclusions contained carbohydrate at 28 h after infection. In contrast to the untreated preparations, in which the number of the carbohydrate-positive inclusions gradually decreased, in the 5FU-treated cells all the inclusions retained carbohydrate and were stained with lugol [Becker, unpublished]. Treatment with antimetabolites caused a change in the degree of branching of the carbohydrate which stained blue, instead of brown, with iodine [Blyth and Reeve, cited in Collier, 1973].

c) Effect of Phlorizin

Phlorizin is an inhibitor of the phosphorylase which is responsible for the conversion of glycogen to glucose-phosphate. Addition of 100 μg/ml of phlorizin to *C. trachomatis* (TE55)-infected FL cells had no effect on the developmental cycle of the agent. The increase in the number of glycogen-positive inclusions was the same as in untreated cells, but the degradation of the carbohydrate was prevented and all the inclusions retained the carbohydrate at the end of the growth cycle [Becker, unpublished]. This result suggested that the degradation of glycogen to glucose-phosphate was not an essential step in the developmental cycle of the agent, and in the absence of glycogen utilization the developmental cycle was unaffected.

4. Glycogen Synthetase

Jenkin and Fan [1971] studied glycogen synthetase activity in *C. trachomatis*-infected and uninfected HeLa cells. It was found that infected HeLa cells (with the TW-3 strain) showed a rise in glycogen synthetase activity, with a peak at 48 h post-infection when adenosine diphosphate glucose (ADPG) was used as a substrate. A similar glycogen synthetase activity was found to increase in LGV-infected cells. In uninfected HeLa cells as well as in *C. psittaci* (meningopneumonitis agent)-infected HeLa cells, the glycogen synthetase differed from that of trachoma-infected cells in its inability to utilize ADPG as a substrate. Only uninfected HeLa cells could utilize uridine diphosphate glucose (UDPG) as a substrate. This result demonstrated that *C. trachomatis* contains the genetic information for a specific glycogen synthetase responsible for the synthesis of the glycogen in the inclusion bodies.

F. Lipid Metabolism and Membrane Biosynthesis

1. ^{3}H-Choline Incorporation into Developing Inclusion Bodies

Preliminary studies [BECKER, unpublished] demonstrated that ^{3}H-choline incorporation by uninfected and TE55-infected FL cells was the same. However, when uninfected and infected cells were homogenized and fractionated by centrifugation in sucrose gradients, it was found that radioactive choline was incorporated in the agent's initial (secondary) bodies and later into the agent's e.b. In such infected cells, less ^{3}H-choline was incorporated into the host cell membrane fraction as compared to uninfected cells. The nature of the changes in the lipid metabolism of the infected cells is not known.

2. The Inclusion-Body Limiting Membrane

Electron microscopy of trachoma-infected cells [BERNKOPF *et al.*, 1962a; MITSUI *et al.*, 1964a; KRAMER and GORDON, 1971] demonstrated that the inclusions are surrounded by a distinct membrane. This inclusion limiting membrane increased in size during the developmental cycle of the agent, even in cells in which host cell protein synthesis was inhibited by the alkaloid emetine [BECKER and ASHER, 1972a]. This led to the conclusion that the synthesis of the inclusion body limiting membrane is probably controlled by *C. trachomatis*. Under conditions which inhibit the development of the trachoma agent (e.g. treatment with rifampicin or chloramphenicol) these limiting membranes were not formed. BLYTH *et al.* [1971] isolated the intact inclusion bodies of TRIC agents (HAR-2f and MRC-4f strains) which retained their glycogen-containing matrix. The inclusion bodies banded in CsCl gradient at a density ranging between 1.65 and 1.68 g/ml. These experiments indicated that the inclusion body membrane might be an integral structure of the developing agent.

3. The Membranes of the Initial and Elementary Bodies

Electron microscopic studies [KRAMER and GORDON, 1971] revealed the presence of a membrane around the initial (secondary) bodies present in the inclusion bodies of the chlamydial agent. The demonstration of secondary bodies which assumed forms of prokaryotic cells in binary fission (fig. 4) suggested that the synthesis of the secondary body membrane continued until two daughter particles were formed. The finding [BECKER, unpublished] that radioactive choline is incorporated into *C. trachomatis* (TE 55) e.b. suggested an active synthesis of the initial body limiting membrane.

G. Cell Wall Synthesis

The formation of initial bodies in the developing trachoma inclusion bodies was accompanied by the synthesis of rigid cell walls as previously demonstrated for *C. psittaci* by JENKIN [1960]. Electron microscopic studies [BERNKOPF *et al.*, 1962a] showed that the formation of initial bodies was inhibited by penicillin, an inhibitor of cell wall synthesis. Electron microscopy of the developing chlamydial inclusions [BERNKOPF *et al.*, 1962a; BECKER *et al.*, 1963; KRAMER and GORDON, 1971] suggested two stages of cell wall synthesis: (a) during the formation of secondary bodies and (b) during the formation of elementary bodies. The cell wall around the newly formed elementary body was found to be loose and remote from the cell membrane. Later, when maturation of the e.b. occurred, the cell wall was tightly attached to the cell membrane. The molecular basis of these processes is not yet known.

The studies on the molecular processes involved in the development of *C. trachomatis* e.b. into initial bodies and finally into the new e.b. progeny are still missing some basic information. The fate of the e.b. cell wall after the initiation of its development in the host cell cytoplasm, as well as the relationship between the e.b. cell membrane and the inclusion body limiting membrane, have not been studied yet. Further research on the transcriptional and translational processes in the developing inclusions is necessary before the mechanisms of trachoma development will be fully elucidated.

VII. Antibiotics against *C. trachomatis* and Trachoma

Due to the prokaryotic nature of *C. trachomatis*, antibiotics which have antibacterial properties also affect the development of the agents, provided they can pass through the host cell membrane. BIETTI and WERNER [1967], TARIZZO and NATAF [1970, 1971] and JAWETZ [1969] summarized the information available on drugs and antibiotics (11 sulfa compounds and 20 antibiotics) which were studied for their antitrachoma activity. The mode of antitrachoma activity of drugs and antibiotics which belong to several groups will be discussed.

A. Mode of Action of Antitrachoma Drugs

1. Sulfonamides

a) Effect on Development of the Trachoma Agent

The *C. trachomatis* (TRIC) agents were found to be sensitive to sulfonamide [T'ANG *et al.*, 1957; GRAYSTON *et al.*, 1960; WERNER, 1961; BERNKOPF *et al.*, 1962b; KURNOSOVA and LENKEVICH, 1964]. Studies by BERNKOPF *et al.* [1962a] demonstrated that the drug sulfanilamido-3 phenyl-2-pyrazole (orisul) did not completely inhibit the development of *C. trachomatis* (TE55 strain) in FL cells even at a concentration of 100 μg/ml. Small vacuoles developed which contained a small number of RNA-containing particles. However, the inhibitory effect of the drug could not be reversed. Lower concentrations of the drug did not prevent the development of infectious e. b. in the inclusion bodies (fig. 10).

Complete inhibition was observed when the drug was added during the first 12 h after infection. When added at 20 and 32 h after infection, the inhibitory effect was only partial.

b) Mode of Action of Sulfa Drugs

COLON and MOULDER [1958] and COLON [1960] reported on the presence

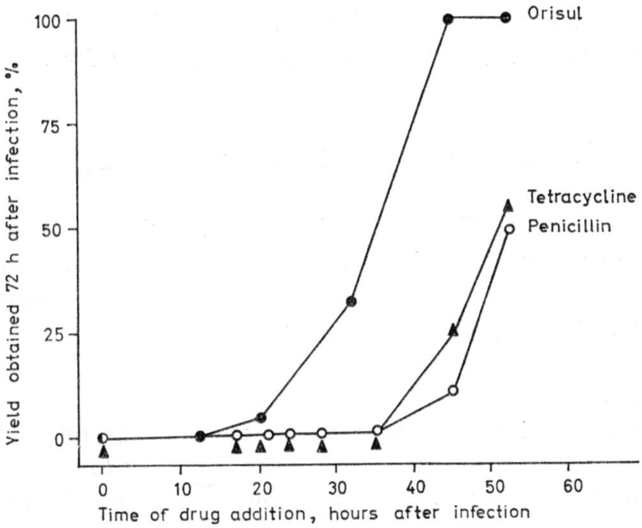

Fig. 10. Effect of penicillin, tetracycline and orisul, added at different intervals after infection, on a trachoma agent in FL cells. The cell cultures were infected with the TE55 strain of trachoma. Penicillin (100 units/ml), tetracycline (0.1 μg/ml) and orisul (10 μg/ml) were added to the culture medium at different time intervals after infection, and the cultures were reincubated for 72 h at 37 °C. The cells were treated in an ultrasonic disintegrator and the yield of infective particles was determined. Orisul = sulfanilamido-3-phenyl-2-pyrazole. From BERNKOPF *et al.* [1962b].

of folic acid synthesizing enzyme in e.b. of *C. psittaci* and the synthesis of folinic acid in tissues infected by the agent. The *C. trachomatis* agents were found to be inhibited [JAWETZ, 1964] most probably because the sulfa drugs blocked the incorporation of para-aminobenzoic acid (PABA) into the folic acid molecule. The inhibitory effect of the drug sulfanilamido-3 phenyl-2-pyrazole (at a concentration of 10 μg/ml) on the T'ang (TE55) strain in FL cells was reversed by addition of 1 μg/ml PABA, 10 μg/ml folinic acid or 100 μg/ml folic acid to the culture medium.

c) Mutations to Sulfonamide-Resistant Trachoma Strains

JOHNSTON *et al.* [1962] reported that treatment of *C. trachomatis* (TW-29 strain)-infected embryonated eggs with sulfadiazine resulted in the emergence of a mutant which was resistant to 5 mg/egg of the drug. SHIAO *et al.* [1967] found that two strains (ND-3 and TW-180) were resistant to sulfadiazine (were not affected by 10 mg/egg). Also, the TW-3 antigenic group of strains showed a tendency to be more resistant than the TW-1 group.

2. Inhibitors of Folic Acid Metabolism

The studies on the effect of sulfa drugs on *C. trachomatis* agents demonstrated the importance of folic acid metabolism in the developmental cycle of the agents. Hence, other inhibitors which are capable of impairing these processes might also prevent trachoma development.

a) Aminopterin

BERNKOPF *et al.* [1962a] demonstrated that aminopterin inhibited the development of the T'ang (TE55) strain of *C. trachomatis* at a concentration of 1 μg/ml. This inhibitory effect was completely reversed by 10 μg/ml of folinic acid.

b) Trimethoprim

Trimethoprim was found to inhibit the formylation of met-t-RNA_F required for the initiation of peptide bond synthesis in bacteria [SHIH *et al.*, 1966]. The inhibitor prevents the transfer of a formyl group from folic acid to the acceptor tRNA. It was found that trimethoprim inhibited the growth of several trachoma strains [REEVE *et al.*, 1968] whereas leucovorin reversed the effect. These results might indicate that the *C. trachomatis* agent contains a dihydrofolate reductase activity. Similarly, it was found [BECKER *et al.*, 1971] that trimethoprim, at a concentration of 1.0 μg/ml, inhibited the formation of 90% of *C. trachomatis* (TE55) e.b., while at a concentration of 100 μg/ml trimethoprim, trachoma development was completely prevented. The inhibitor was found to completely stop the synthesis of trachoma RNA [BECKER, unpublished].

B. Mode of Antitrachoma Action of Antibiotics

1. Penicillin

a) Inhibition of Trachoma Development

Even in large doses, penicillin failed to cause complete suppression of the development of the agent. At a concentration of 0.1 units/ml of penicillin

G and V, the vacuoles which appeared in the cytoplasm of the infected cells at 24–48 h contained large irregularly-formed masses which stained an uneven bluish-red with Giemsa. Preparations stained with acridine orange and examined by fluorescence microscopy revealed that these structures took on a red color (RNA type). In later stages of development, green staining material (DNA type) was seen lying next to and around the masses. In the presence of 0.1 units/ml a few particles of elementary body size also appeared in a small number of the inclusions. They became much more numerous at a concentration of 0.01 units/ml of penicillin. At this concentration, many mature inclusion bodies were observed. In a number of experiments, *C. trachomatis*-infected penicillin-treated cultures were examined for the presence of infective particles after 72 h of incubation. For this purpose, sufficient penicillinase was added to the culture medium to degrade the antibiotic. No evidence of infectivity was observed when penicillin in concentrations of 0.1 or more units/ml had been added to the cultures immediately after infection. In the presence of 0.01 units/ml of penicillin many infective particles developed in the inclusions, but only 50% or less of the infectivity in untreated controls was reached. Even at this low concentration, penicillin showed some obvious inhibitory effect. The action of penicillin, when added at different intervals after infection, was also examined. Penicillin, at a concentration of 100 units/ml, completely prevented the appearance of infective particles when added as late as 28 h. Addition of the drug 35, 45 and 52 h after infection gave rise to 1, 10 and 50%, respectively, of the maximal e.b. yield of the controls (fig. 10) [BERNKOPF *et al.*, 1962a].

b) Mode of Action

Penicillin interferes with the synthesis of cell walls within the developing inclusion bodies [BERNKOPF *et al.*, 1962b; GILKES *et al.*, 1958; KRAMER and GORDON, 1971]. JAWETZ [1964] emphasized the analogy of penicillin inhibition of TRIC agent to its effect on bacterial cell wall synthesis [PERKINS, 1969].

2. Tetracyclines

The studies on the effect of tetracyclines on the agents of trachoma were summarized by JAWETZ [1964] and by TARIZZO and NABLI [1967]. Oxytetracycline and tetracycline were found to be most effective in inhibiting the *C. trachomatis* (TE55) agent [BERNKOPF *et al.*, 1962a]. Tetracycline hydro-

Table V. Reversal of trachoma agent inhibition by antitrachoma drugs

Drug removed, h post-infection	Drug			
	rifampicin	rifamycin 33	achromycin	erythromycin
	progeny of trachoma agent, PFU/ml			
5	2.0×10^7	3.0×10^7	3.0×10^7	2.0×10^7
8	1.2×10^6	8.0×10^6	6.0×10^6	3.5×10^6
12	3.0×10^5	2.0×10^6	4.0×10^6	4.5×10^6
24	0	1.0×10^6	4.0×10^6	4.0×10^6
28	0	2.5×10^6	2.0×10^6	1.0×10^6
48	0	0	4.5×10^5	4.0×10^5
72				
with drugs	0	0	0	0

From BECKER *et al.* [1971; p. 18].

chloride at a concentration of 8 μg/ml completely inhibited (99.99% inhibition) the development of trachoma strains other than the T'ang (TE55) strain. However, at concentrations up to 32 μg/ml of tetracycline, all the tested strains were inhibited [JAWETZ, 1962a, b].

The intracellular site of action of this group of antibiotics is at the ribosome level [WEISSBLUM and DAVIES, 1968]. The synthesis of proteins was inhibited due to interference of the antibiotic with the binding of aminoacyl-tRNA to the ribosome-mRNA complexes. The inhibitory effect of tetracyclines on trachoma was reversed after removal of the antibiotic (achromycin) from the medium of *C. trachomatis* (TE55)-infected cultures [BECKER *et al.*, 1971]. This result indicated that the antibiotics are inhibitory only when present in the infected cells (table V).

3. Chloramphenicol

Complete inhibition of *C. trachoma* (TE55) was achieved at a concentration of 1.0 μg/ml [BERNKOPF *et al.*, 1962a]. The inhibition was due to the inhibition of protein synthesis. It was also found that treatment of trachoma (TE55)-infected cells with chloramphenicol did not prevent the initial synthesis of the precursor for ribosomal RNA molecules but inhibited the conversion of the precursor molecules to mature ribosomal RNA [GUTTER and BECKER, 1972].

4. Rifampicin

a) Effect on Trachoma Development

Rifampicin, a semisynthetic antibiotic (fig. 11), inhibits the development of trachoma agent at a concentration of 0.01 μg/ml. The agents of inclusion conjunctivitis, lymphogranuloma venereum and psittacosis also are inhibited by the antibiotic [BECKER and ZAKAY-RONES, 1969; BECKER *et al.*, 1969a, 1970, 1971; BECKER, 1971a, b, 1972a, b; NABLI, 1971].

The effect of rifampicin on the growth cycle of the TE55 strain of trachoma was studied (fig. 12). It was found [BECKER and ZAKAY-RONES, 1969] that the initial effect of the antibiotic is prevention of formation of the e. b. progeny and the second effect is decrease in the amount of the infecting e. b. which stayed in the infected cells but did not develop.

b) Irreversibility of Rifampicin Inhibition

It was demonstrated [BECKER *et al.*, 1971] that rifampicin irreversibly inhibited the development of the trachoma agent (TE55) in cell cultures. Removal of the antibiotic from the medium of the infected cells did not result in the recovery of infective e. b. progeny (table V).

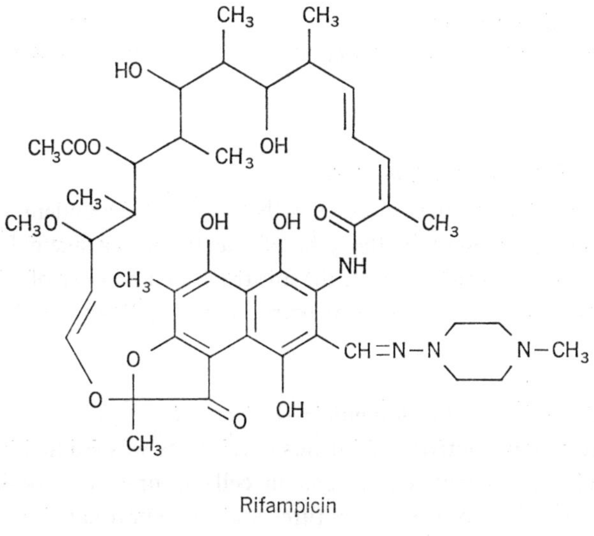

Fig. 11. The chemical composition of rifampicin.

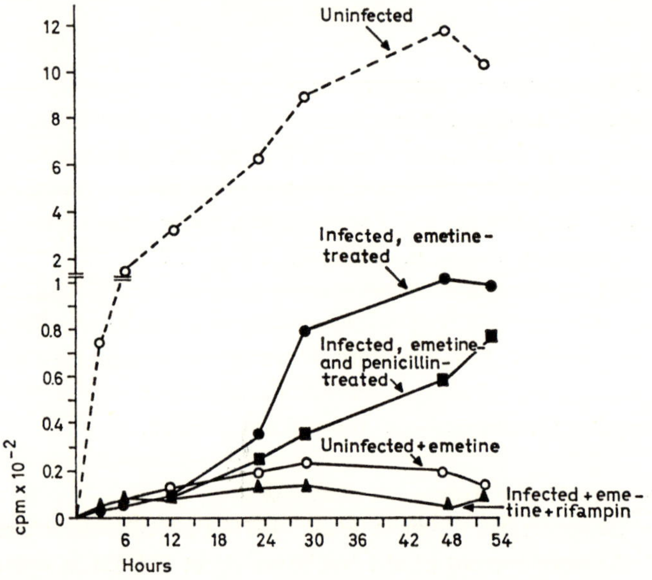

Fig. 12. Effect of rifampicin and penicillin on trachoma protein synthesis. Emetine-treated, trachoma-infected cells were labeled with 0.5 μCi of ^{3}H-leucine per milliliter. Some of the infected, emetine-treated cultures were treated with penicillin (100 μg/ml) or rifampicin (1 μg/ml). Uninfected cells and emetine-treated, uninfected cells served as controls. The radioactivity in the cells and in the trachoma proteins was determined at different time intervals. ○---○ = Uninfected, untreated; ○——○ = uninfected, emetine-treated; ● = infected, emetine-treated; ▲ = infected, emetine- and rifampicin-treated; ■ = infected, emetine- and penicillin-treated. From BECKER and ASHER [1972b].

c) Mode of Action of Rifampicin

The antibiotic molecules interact with the DNA-dependent RNA polymerase molecules present in the e.b. of the trachoma agent [SAROV and BECKER, 1971a, b]. In this respect, the antitrachoma activity of rifampicin is identical to its mode of action in prokaryotic cells [WEHRLI and STAEHELIN, 1969].

d) Inhibitory Effects by Rifampicin Derivatives

The antitrachoma activity of various derivatives was studied in trachoma agent-infected embryonated eggs and in cell cultures. Compound 33 was found to be effective both in cell cultures and in embryonated eggs. Rifamycin SV affected trachoma development in cultured cells but not in embryonated eggs. Similar results were obtained with derivatives No. 11, 18 and 26 of rifamycin SV [BECKER *et al.*, 1970].

To determine whether rifamycin derivatives had an antitrachoma activity, in addition to the anti-RNA polymerase activity, the effect of rifamycin derivatives, which lacked the ability to inhibit RNA polymerase, on trachoma development was studied. It was found that the derivative 8-0-acetylrifamycin A inhibited *C. trachomatis* (TE55) development in FL cells, indicating the presence of a secondary inhibitory site in the rifampicin molecule.

5. Streptovaricin

This antibiotic [MIZUNO *et al.*, 1968] resembles the antibiotic rifamycin in its chemical structure. The effect of the antibiotic on the development of the trachoma agent was therefore studied. Streptovaricin was found to be toxic to embryonated eggs, and hence it was not possible to study its effect on trachoma strains, which can be propagated only in embryonated eggs. However, streptovaricin inhibited the development of the *C. trachomatis* (TE55) agent in cultured cells at concentrations of 1 to 10 μg/ml, depending on the type of cell culture. The inhibitory effect was reversible, and the agent developed inclusion bodies after the removal of the antibiotic [BECKER, unpublished].

6. Macrolides

This group of antibiotics (which includes erythromycin, oleandomycin, spyromycin, tylosin and carbomycin) inhibits the formation of peptide bonds at the ribosomal level. POLLARD and TANAMI [1962] found that tylosine tartrate inhibited trachoma development in cell cultures. JAWETZ [1962a, b] found that the same drug inhibited trachoma development in embryonated eggs but only at high concentrations (500 μg/ml).

7. Hydroxyurea

Treatment of *C. trachomatis* (TE55)-infected FL cells with different concentrations of hydroxyurea resulted in various inhibitory effects on the agent's developmental cycle. At a concentration of 10^{-2} M, hydroxyurea prevented trachoma development in an irreversible way. At lower concentrations (10^{-3} M to 5×10^{-4} M) the development of the inclusion bodies was not affected, but the formation of e.b. was prevented. Upon removal of the drug the formation of e.b. was initiated. Hydroxyurea inhibits the synthesis of *C. trachomatis* DNA [ROSENKRANZ *et al.*, 1973].

8. Metabolic Analogs

The effect of 5-fluorodeoxycytidine on the development of the *C. trachomatis* (T'ang strain) agent was studied by SHARON and POLLARD [1963]. The development of the agent was inhibited by the analog, especially when added 12–16 h after infection. Addition of thymidine to the treated cultures reversed the inhibitory effect. Treatment of *C. trachomatis* (TE55 strain) with 5-fluorouracil (FU) affected the synthesis of RNA in the developing agent. Addition of 5-fluoro-2-deoxyuridine (FUDR) affected the agent's DNA synthesis [POLLARD and TANAMI, 1962].

9. Antibiotics Inhibitory at High Concentrations

SOWA and RACE [1971] reported that neomycin and streptomycin, when used at high concentrations and for prolonged periods, not only inhibited the bacterial contaminants present in the samples obtained from trachomatous conjunctivae, but also diminished the chance of isolating *C. trachomatis* agents at the first passage. Sensitivity of trachoma strains to streptomycin was also noted.

C. Drugs and Antibiotics in the Treatment of Trachoma Patients

JAWETZ [1969] summarized in his review the clinical use of drugs in the treatment of *C. trachomatis* (TRIC) infections of the eye. In spite of therapeutic attempts since then, JAWETZ [1971] maintained the idea that treatment of trachoma patients 'favors suppression of the organism and reduces manifest disease, but treatment rarely eliminates the infectious agent completely'. Recent therapeutic trials were summarized by TARIZZO and NATAF [1970, 1971].

1. Treatment with Sulfonamides

a) Long-Acting Sulfonamides

Sulfonamides were used in the treatment of trachoma infections either locally or systemically, using several cycles of treatment with adequate supervision of the patients. Therefore, long-acting sulfonamides which are slowly excreted might be advantageous in simplifying and enhancing the efficacy of treatment [Bietti *et al.*, 1967b].

b) Sulfonamide Treatment in Endemic Areas

Tarizzo and Nataf [1970] summarized the studies in which sulfa drugs were used for treatment of trachoma in patients living in endemic areas. They concluded that 'most of the available evidence, notwithstanding some of its inadequacy and some of the more skeptical reports, indicate that sulfonamides are effective against trachoma in individual cases and that their use would be cheap and a relatively simple way to deal with the problem where the disease is endemic.' Their introduction in large quantities in communities with a low educational level, as is often the case in areas where trachoma is highly prevalent, may present an added health hazard because of the possibility of side reactions requiring adequate supervision. Mitsui *et al.* [1963] found that sulfonamides given by intramuscular injections and not by oral treatment were adequate for treatment of patients in rural areas.

2. Treatment with Antibiotics

Ostler *et al.* [1971] and Dawson *et al.* [1971] studied the effect of orally administered doxycycline in comparison to oral tetracycline in a group of selected American Indian children. The results indicated that the incidence of clinical trachoma diminished at a similar rate in both treated and control groups. Tarizzo and Nataf [1970] summarized the studies on treatment with tetracyclines of trachoma patients in various endemic areas. The antibiotics (tetracycline, oxytetracycline or chlortetracycline-1 % suspension) were applied locally to the conjunctival sacs of trachoma patients during trachoma control projects in 21 countries. The conclusion [Tarizzo and Nataf, 1970] was 'that large scale antibiotic treatment of trachoma can significantly contribute to the solution of this important public health problem where the disease is endemic.' Gupta *et al.* [1968] suggested the use of tetracyclines for the treatment of trachoma patients in endemic areas.

3. Doxycycline Treatment of Patients with Chronic Trachoma

Hoshiwara *et al.* [1973] studied the efficiency of daily treatment of children with mild, chronic trachoma using doxycycline (a slowly excreted tetracycline; 28 doses of 2.5–4 mg/kg during a 40-day period). The doxycycline-treated children improved markedly as compared to those who received placebo. The authors suggested that one dose per day of doxycycline should be considered for mass treatment in endemic areas. A single course of doxycycline produced striking clinical improvement, but did not eradicate the infectious agent from the tissues.

D. Effect of Interferon on Experimental Trachoma Infections

1. Effect of Interferon on Trachoma Development

Hanna *et al.* [1966, 1967], Vilcek and Jahiel [1970] and Kazar *et al.* [1971] demonstrated that the development of trachoma agents was inhibited in interferon-treated cells. The mode of action of interferon is not yet known. Mordhorst *et al.* [1967] demonstrated inhibition of trachoma development *in ovo* by concentrated chick interferon.

2. Effect of Interferon Inducers on Infection

The effect of interferon inducers on experimental trachoma lesions in rabbits was studied [Oh *et al.*, 1971]. Three interferon inducers were studied: poly I:C, typhoid endotoxin and live Newcastle disease virus. Intravenous injections of the interferon inducers induced varying amounts of interferon in the blood and aqueous humor, but no correlation with the degree of lesion suppression was found. It was suggested that some factors other than interferon play a role in the suppression of ocular lesions produced by the trachoma agent in rabbits. Kazar *et al.* [1971] studied the effect of poly I:C on experimental infections with aerosolized *C. trachomatis*. Intranasal injection with 100 μg of poly I:C, 24 h after intravenous injection of 200 μg poly I:C, did not protect the mice from infection.

VIII. Immunobiology

In a review on the serology and immunology of trachoma, BERNKOPF *et al.* [1966a] summarized the development and usefulness of immunological techniques (complement fixation, fluorescent antibodies, indirect hemagglutination, immunodiffusion, mouse toxin protection and skin tests) in the study of *C. trachomatis*. The use of these techniques made possible investigations on the immunological responses to the trachoma agent in humans and animals.

A. Immunological Responses to the Trachoma Agent

1. Local Antibodies in Humans

a) Detection of Antibodies

Analysis of the conjunctival sac fluids from trachoma patients by the indirect fluorescent antibody technique revealed the presence of immunoglobulins with specificity for the trachoma agent [BERNKOPF *et al.*, 1966b], thus indicating that the presence of trachoma antigens in the infected eyes induced the synthesis of local antibodies. Antibodies to the trachoma agent were also demonstrated in trachoma patients from Saudi Arabia [MCCOMB and NICHOLS, 1969, 1970] at high prevalence. JAWETZ *et al.* [1971] demonstrated antitrachoma antibodies in tears of 11% of school children with active trachoma (16 out of 134 children). A lower incidence was found in patients with chronic mild trachoma and a higher rate in adults with sporadic TRIC infections (50%; 8/16 adults).

b) Characterization of the Antitrachoma Antibodies

Analysis of the antitrachoma antibodies in secretions obtained from trachoma-infected eyes demonstrated the presence of both IgG and IgA globulins. The IgA antibodies were present in lower concentrations than IgG antibodies [JAWETZ *et al.*, 1971]. These authors also reported that IgG antibodies were present in 50% of acute TRIC infections in San Francisco, indicating a correlation between the prevalence of the infectious trachoma agents and the specific antibodies. HATHAWAY and PETERS [1971] demonstrated the presence of IgE globulins, in addition to IgG and IgA, in the eye secretions of trachoma patients [PETERS *et al.*, 1969]. The IgE antibody in the eye secretions reacted with the homologous trachoma antigen.

COLLIER *et al.* [1972] found IgG and IgA antibodies in the conjunctival secretions of young Gambian children. Antibodies were almost never present in the absence of follicles, but the titers were unrelated to the degree of follicular hyperplasia.

c) The Role of Antitrachoma Antibodies in the Eyes

HATHAWAY and PETERS [1971] speculated that IgG antibodies could play a blocking role in preventing the attachment of IgE antibodies and inhibiting the subsequent immediate hypersensitivity reactions. The question if IgA and IgG antibodies in eye secretions play a role in protecting the eyes from trachoma infection has not yet been solved.

2. Local Antibodies in Experimental Infections of Animals

a) Antibody Response to Trachoma Antigens in Guinea Pig Eyes

ZAKAY-RONES *et al.* [1969] immunized guinea pigs eyes topically with homogenates of purified trachoma elementary bodies. Antitrachoma antibodies were detected in the eyes. It was also possible to detect in the conjunctiva antibody-producing cells which reacted with trachoma antigen. These cells infiltrated into the conjunctiva as a result of the administration of trachoma antigen. MURRAY and CHARBONNET [1971] demonstrated that guinea pigs infected in their eyes with the inclusion conjunctivitis (Gp-ic) agent developed noncomplement-fixing, antisecretory IgA antibodies in the eye secretions. The results demonstrated that immunoglobulins can be induced in guinea pigs as a result of the introduction of specific chlamydial antigens.

b) Local Antibodies in Monkeys' Eyes

Owl monkeys *(Aotus trivirgatus)* were used by MURRAY *et al.* [1971] as a model system for the study of trachoma infections. These monkeys are readily infected on the conjunctiva by *C. trachomatis* agents and develop the manifestations of the disease. Antitrachoma antibodies in eye secretions developed concomitantly with the infection. Marked resistance to reinfection was demonstrable with homologous and heterologous *C. trachomatis* strains. Topical instillations of killed *C. trachomatis* antigens (HAR-36 strain) to the conjunctival sac of owl monkeys, which had no antibodies in the eye secretions, did not stimulate the appearance of antitrachoma antibodies. However, when challenged, these monkeys had inclusion rates lower than the non-immunized ones [McComb *et al.*, 1971]. It was concluded that increased antibody titers in the eye secretions were associated with a diminution in inclusion rates after challenge.

Wang and Grayston [1971b] studied, with the aid of a micro-immunofluorescence test, the antibody response against different types of trachoma agents in the serum and eye secretions of monkeys undergoing experimental trachoma eye infections. Local eye antibodies appeared in the secretions from infected eyes in hyperimmune monkeys. The trachoma antibodies were predominantly IgG but IgA antibodies were also found.

3. Antitrachoma Antibodies in Human Sera

a) Serum Antibodies in Trachoma Patients

The antitrachoma antibody titer was found to gradually increase within 7 weeks after infection with the trachoma agent [Bernkopf *et al.*, 1964]. Analysis of the antitrachoma antibody species in the sera of trachoma patients demonstrated IgG and IgA globulins. IgM antibodies were not detected even in early sera specimens taken within 4 days of the onset of clinical eye signs [Jawetz *et al.*, 1971]. Complement-fixing antibodies to chlamydial agents were detected in humans with genital and ocular infections and with Reiter's disease [Barwell *et al.*, 1967]. Schachter [1971] also reported on the presence of group-specific antibodies in patients with Reiter's syndrome.

b) Serum Antibodies in Experimental Animals

Antibodies to LGV appeared in the serum of monkeys within 1 week following intraocular infection or intramuscular injection of the LGV agent; the antibodies were exclusively IgG. None of the 8 monkeys studied showed evidence of IgM or IgA [Isa, 1971]. Wang and Grayston [1971b] demonstrated that in monkeys undergoing experimental eye infection, IgM antibodies appeared first in the serum and later were replaced by IgG antibodies. After reinfection with a new type, IgM antibodies to the new type appeared, but were not seen following reinfections with the same type. IgM antibodies were found only in the serum and not in the eye secretions. This finding agrees with the observation that topical immunization of guinea pigs' eyes induced the appearance of IgM antibodies in the serum [ZAKAY-RONES *et al.*, 1969]. Serum antibodies were also demonstrated in monkeys which were topically immunized with killed trachoma antigens [MCCOMB *et al.*, 1971].

c) Effect of Route of Immunization on the Antibodies in Guinea Pigs' Eyes

Intramuscular inoculation of trachoma antigens [ZAKAY-RONES *et al.*, 1969] or intraperitoneal injection of Gp-ic organisms [MURRAY and CHARBONNET, 1971] into guinea pigs did not stimulate the formation of secretory antibodies in the eyes of immunized animals. Only serum antibodies were detected.

4. Delayed Hypersensitivity

a) Role in the Pathogenesis of the Disease

Studies on the prevention of experimental trachoma in monkeys by immunization [GRAYSTON, 1967; WANG and GRAYSTON, 1967a, b] demonstrated that chronic trachoma with pannus developed after (a) reinfections or relapses, or (b) after immunization with an inadequate vaccine [KUO *et al.*, 1971b, c]. These results suggested that delayed hypersensitivity plays an important role in the pathogenesis of trachoma.

b) In Humans

Injection of a suspension of purified, undamaged elementary bodies into humans elicited positive skin reactions in trachomatous patients and also in some nontrachomatous individuals. Among nontrachomatous subjects, the degree of reaction intensity increased with age, possibly due to infection with other chlamydial agents [BIETTI *et al.*, 1967a]. Experiments on skin tests in trachoma patients were summarized by BERNKOPF *et al.* [1966a].

c) Experimental Delayed Hypersensitivity

Experiments were carried out by BIETTI *et al.* [1967a] to reproduce in rabbits, immunized against trachoma antigens, a delayed reaction, employing different preparations of trachoma antigens. No delayed reaction was demonstrable. KUO *et al.* [1971b] utilized guinea pigs, sensitized with inactivated trachoma organisms, for the study of delayed hypersensitivity to *C. tracho-*

matis. It was found that trachoma allergen was a heat-stable protein. Heated *C. trachomatis* (TW-5, TW-3), LGV and psittacosis (Cal-10 strain) organisms showed a similar reaction by dermal hypersensitivity. Further studies [Kuo *et al.*, 1971c] demonstrated that, in guinea pigs sensitized subcutaneously with *C. trachomatis* e.b., the peripheral blood lymphocytes reacted *in vitro* by incorporation of tritiated thymidine when treated with trachoma allergen. *C. trachomatis* strains could be differentiated from *C. psittaci* by this test but not from other *C. trachomatis* strains.

d) Induction of Delayed Hypersensitivity in Monkeys

Vaccines were prepared from purified *C. trachomatis* elementary bodies (G-1 TRIC agent) by (a) treatment for 2 h with trypsin to produce cell walls, (b) heating to 60 °C for 30 min and (c) extraction of lipids. Monkeys *(Macaca cyclopis)* were immunized with the three vaccines [Grayston *et al.*, 1971] and challenged with the G-1 strain. It was found that the immunized monkeys suffered relatively severe illness which included development of pannus and spontaneous cross-infection to the uninoculated eye. A similar enhancement in clinical response of monkeys to a heterologous challenge was previously reported by Mordhorst [1967a, b].

e) Differentiation of Chlamydial Agents by a Delayed-Type Hypersensitivity Test

Kassira [1971] utilized the skin test in sensitized guinea pigs for the differentiation of chlamydial antigens, using reaction size as a measure. It was found that the homologous test systems resulted in larger reactions.

B. Characterization of Antitrachoma Antibodies

1. Neutralizing Antibodies

a) Neutralization of Homologous Strains

Reeve and Graham [1962] demonstrated that specific antibodies neutralized the infectivity of trachoma elementary bodies. Further studies [Graham and Layton, 1971] revealed that sera prepared against strain MU-16 of *C. trachomatis* contained antibodies that neutralized the infectivity of the homologous strain for Vero cells but not the infectivity of a heterologous strain, HAR-2. Similarly, Zakay-Rones and Becker [1971] demonstrated that a low titer of neutralizing antibodies for homologous *C. trachomatis* strains was present in hyperimmune rabbit sera. The extent of neutralization was not enhanced by the addition of anti-γ-globulin. MOGG *et al.* [1971] also reported on low-titer neutralizing antibodies in the IgM and IgG globulin fractions of immunized rabbits.

b) Neutralization of Heterologous Strains

ZAKAY-RONES and BECKER [1971] demonstrated that antibodies were found in the serum of immunized rabbits; the serum reacted with heterologous trachoma elementary bodies in the presence of anti-γ-globulin. Even under these conditions, the heterologous neutralizing antibodies neutralized only $10^{2.5}$ to $10^{4.0}$ EID_{50} of *C. trachomatis*.

2. Antibodies to Specific Antigens

a) Antibodies to Group-Specific Antigen

Studies by GRAHAM and LAYTON [1971] demonstrated that antibodies to the group-specific antigens (determined by the complement-fixation test) appeared 5–6 days after the injection into rabbits of a single dose of partially purified e.b. obtained from heavily infected egg yolks. These antibodies persisted in the rabbits for a prolonged period of time. MOGG *et al.* [1971], using the complement-fixation technique to measure chlamydial group-specific antibodies, had found that after the initial antigen dose, the average antibody titer in the sera of the immunized rabbits rose sharply during the first week, reached maximum at the 4th week and then declined rapidly. After each injection, antibodies were present in both IgM and IgG globulins. MOGG *et al.* [1971] indicated that in the rabbit the immunological response to chlamydial antigens resembled the antibody induction by rickettsiae and gram-negative bacteria. Antibodies were present in trachoma (TW-3)-immunized rabbit serum which reacted with a carbohydrate fraction extracted from trachoma organisms [DHIR *et al.*, 1972].

b) Antibodies to Cell Wall Antigens

PHILIP *et al.* [1967] reported that cell wall antigens were useful in determining serological relationships between LGV and some *C. trachomatis* (TRIC) strains. Treatment of *C. trachomatis* (HAR-3) elementary bodies with neuraminidase enhanced the antigenic and immunogenic properties of the preparations [PETERS, 1967].

C. Experimental Immunization against Trachoma

1. Immunological Responses to Trachoma Vaccines in Animals

a) Guinea Pigs

Injection of purified trachoma e.b. into guinea pigs resulted in an antibody response. Formalin treatment of the e.b. lessened the antibody response, whereas adjuvants improved it [BERNKOPF and NISHMI, 1967]. MURRAY and CHARBONNET [1971] inoculated formalin-killed Gp-ic organisms into guinea pigs to study the role of immunization in the protection of eyes against infection with the homologous agent. It was found that the immunized animals showed no immunity to subsequent conjunctival challenge with live (Gp-ic strain) e.b., although a high titer of CF antibodies was demonstrable. BLYTH [1967] had found that vaccination by killed trachoma e.b. injected intracutaneously or intravenously did not protect the guinea pigs against skin injection of live organisms.

b) Owl Monkeys

Immunization of owl monkeys with purified, killed trachoma antigens (strain HAR-36) by topical instillation into the conjunctival sacs of 12 monkeys was studied by McCOMB *et al.* [1971]. It was found that when the titer of antibodies increased in immunized monkeys, which were serum-negative prior to vaccination, the monkeys had lower inclusion rates than did the controls. It was also found that many monkeys had antibodies to the trachoma agent in the serum as well as in the eye secretions. Resistance to an infectious challenge of 2,000 EID_{50} of *C. trachomatis* (HAR-36 strain) was related to the initial antibody levels in the monkeys.

2. Other Species of Monkeys

a) Dissemination of Infective Trachoma Elementary Bodies in Baboons

COLLIER and SMITH [1967] demonstrated that 5 min after subcutaneous injection of baboons with live e.b. the agent was recovered from the site of injection. After 4 days, the regional lymph nodes contained infectious particles, which remained present for a month. During this period, low titers of infectious particles were detected in the spleen. Intravenously inoculated e.b. were detected in lymph nodes within 2 days after injection, and the spleen increased in weight. This study provided information regarding the distribution of e.b. in the body after injection and also demonstrated that live e.b. developed in tissue cells. Heat inactivation or formalin treatment of *C. trachomatis* e.b. destroyed the antigenicity of the agent [COLLIER *et al.*, 1967].

b) Importance of Content of Elementary Bodies in the Vaccine

GRAYSTON *et al.* [1971] immunized monkeys *(Macaca cyclopis)* with sucrose gradient- and genetron-purified *C. trachomatis* (strain TW-5, type B) at three concentrations: 4×10^9, 4×10^8 and 4×10^7 elementary bodies per sample. All monkeys, including unimmunized controls, were challenged in one eye with the TW-1 (type B) strain and in the other with the TW-3 (type C) strain of *C. trachomatis,* partially purified e.b. from infected yolk sacs ($10^{3.5}$ EID_{50}). It was found that protection was afforded against the homologous strain at the first challenge, only if the vaccine contained 10^9 particles. No effect on the heterologous strain was noted. A second challenge 9 months later with the genetron-purified e.b. vaccine exerted a protective effect. However, the third challenge, 2 years after injection, resulted in an enhanced severity of infection in the animals that had received the vaccine as compared to the controls. Similar results were reported by WANG *et al.* [1967a] and by MORDHORST [1967a, b].

c) Immunization of Monkeys with a Trivalent Vaccine

Injection of 5×10^9 trachoma elementary bodies (made up of equal amounts of each of the three immunological types A, B and C) into monkeys resulted in protection against each of the three trachoma types. At lower concentrations of elementary bodies, the vaccine failed to protect. The disease in monkeys immunized with 5×10^7 elementary bodies was more severe than in the controls [GRAYSTON *et al.*, 1971]. These results demonstrated that immunization with inadequate amounts of antigen might lead to a severe response in the eyes upon infection.

d) Conclusions

The results of experiments by WANG and GRAYSTON [1967a, b] and GRAYSTON *et al.* [1971] suggested: (i) vaccines of at least 10^9 elementary bodies per milliliter are necessary to obtain a protective effect; (ii) vaccination protects against infection with the homologous *C. trachomatis* agent; (iii) the trachoma elementary bodies should be emulsified with mineral oil immediately before vaccination; and (iv) immunization with vaccines containing lower e.b. doses must be prohibited.

3. Immunization of Humans

Preventive vaccination of humans, or the use of vaccination in the treatment of resistant cases of trachoma [TERSKIKH *et al.*, 1967], are still regarded as experimental [TARIZZO and NATAF, 1970]. The above-mentioned studies on the immunization of monkeys might provide the approach to vaccination of humans.

a) Antitrachoma Vaccination Trials in Taiwan

i) Initial studies. Preschool children were immunized with a vaccine containing *C. trachomatis* e.b. (strains TW-1 or a mixture of TW-1 and TW-3) [GRAYSTON *et al.*, 1962; WOOLRIDGE *et al.*, 1967a, b, c]. The vaccine was prepared from infected yolk sacs by the use of trypsin, differential centrifugation and precipitation of egg material with polymyxin, and was mixed with alum prior to administration. At the end of 2 years, the vaccine had reduced trachoma infections by 60%. However, beginning 2.5–3 years after immunization (a year after the booster injection), the protection afforded to the vaccinated children began to disappear, and at the end of 6 years the vaccinated group resembled the unvaccinated ones.

ii) Monovalent and bivalent mineral adjuvant trachoma vaccine. The vaccine consisted of either TW-1 or TW-1 and TW-3 *C. trachomatis* strains which were purified from yolk sac suspensions through DEAE-Sephadex H-50 columns. The purified e.b. were further concentrated, and equal portions of the e.b. suspension and the mineral oil adjuvant (85% Bayol F and 15% Arlacel A) were mixed by circulating from one syringe to another [WOOLRIDGE *et al.*, 1967b]. The results of this study, carried out in children with no evidence of trachoma infections, demonstrated that (i) the bivalent (TW-1 and TW-3) vaccine produced a modest protective effect; (ii) the monovalent (TW-3) vaccine was associated with a considerably higher trachoma rate than the control (placebo-treated) group; (iii) the bivalent vaccine was of low potency because of a low content of elementary bodies, probably due to the inadequate purification technique; and (iv) the monovalent vaccine caused deleterious effects in the vaccinated individuals, probably due to hypersensitivity reactions.

b) Vaccination of Children in Punjab Indian Villages

Studies were carried out by DHIR *et al.* [1967] on the efficacy of two trachoma vaccines: a genetron-purified vaccine containing equal amounts of elementary bodies of two Taiwan *C. trachomatis* strains (TW-3 and TW-5), and a vaccine made of e.b. purified in sucrose gradients. The genetron vaccine contained 2.2×10^9 particles, and the sucrose gradient vaccine contained 1.2×10^9 particles per milliliter. (Nitrogen content was 0.2 mg/ml and 0.34 mg/ml, respectively.) Both vaccines protected against trachoma infections during a period of one year but the protection decreased gradually during this period. At the end of one year, the incidence of trachoma infections in the unimmunized group was 37% while only 10% of the immunized group contracted trachoma.

c) A Field Trial in Saudi Arabia [Nichols *et al.*, 1969]

Children in Saudi Arabia were vaccinated with a formalinized vaccine preparation which contained equal proportions of two *C. trachomatis* strains (TRIC/1/ET/Har-13/OT[Egypt-2] and TRIC/2/SAU/Har-2/OT[SA-2]). The two strains represented the two major types found in Arabia. The content of e.b. in the preparation was estimated on the basis of infectious doses for chick embryos or toxicity for mice. 12% of the children were inclusion-positive at the prevaccination examination. No effect of the vaccine was found on the trachoma attack rates during a period of 24 months, but a reduction in inclusions was observed in the vaccinated children.

d) Antitrachoma Vaccination Trials in Ethiopia

Experiments on the prevention and therapy of trachoma were carried out in Ethiopia by Bietti *et al.* [1963, 1964, 1965, 1968] and Guerra *et al.* [1967, 1971].

i) Preparation of the vaccine. The vaccine used by Bietti *et al.* [1964] was (i) an aqueous vaccine which contained a suspension of elementary bodies in saline to make up a final 100-percent yolk sac pool, (ii) a suspension of equal parts of purified and concentrated elementary bodies in saline and of aluminum (19 mg/ml) to make up a final twofold concentration, and (iii) a suspension of purified and concentrated elementary bodies in saline and oil adjuvant (Arlacel, 1 part, and Bayol F, 9 parts). The vaccine used by Guerra *et al.* [1967] was a purified preparation of elementary bodies of a trachoma strain isolated in Ethiopia (TRIC/EAE/ASM/1960/OT) and cultivated in the yolk sac of embryonated eggs. The yolk sacs were treated with trypsin and ether, and the elementary bodies were purified and concentrated by differential centrifugation [Bietti *et al.*, 1966]. The elementary bodies were resuspended in saline containing 0.02% formalin, which was later neutralized with stoichiometric quantities of sodium metabisulphite. The number of particles in the vaccine were counted by the method of REEVE and TAVERNE [1962]. The batches of the vaccine were standardized according to the number of elementary bodies, DNA and protein contents, and antigenicity [BIETTI *et al.*, 1966]. The vaccine contained 5×10^8 elementary bodies per dose for the initial injection and 2.5×10^8 particles for the second one, which was administered 6 weeks after the first injection. It should be noted that the concentration of e.b. in the vaccine was one-tenth of the concentration that GRAYSTON *et al.* [1971] found to be effective in the immunization of monkeys.

ii) Results of vaccinations. It was concluded [GUERRA *et al.*, 1967] that the activity of the vaccine began to be noticeable 6 months after vaccination and was evident 2.5 years later. The unexpectedly high rate of favorable results in the mock-immunized individuals of groups similar to the vaccinated ones was not explained. Two and one-half years after vaccination, the number of infected or unhealed individuals from the placebo-treated groups was increasing as compared to the vaccinated ones.

iii) Combined vaccination and chemotherapy. GUERRA *et al.* [1971] immunized preschool children by administering 5×10^8 and 2.5×10^8 elementary bodies/ml in two injections 40 days apart, and treated the same children with long-acting sulfonamide. With combined treatment in the 0- to 3-year-old and 4- to 7-year-old groups, an improvement was observed. In contrast to these findings, three field trials on the usefulness of trachoma vaccine in combination with drug therapy failed because of the inability to cure trachoma with tetracycline eye ointment either alone or combined with the trachoma vaccine [WOOLRIDGE *et al.*, 1967a].

e) Vaccinotherapy Studies in USSR

i) Vaccine. TERSKIKH *et al.* [1967] used the Burkham strain of trachoma [isolated from a trachoma patient and cultivated in chick embryo fibroblasts (70–75% infected cells)]. The method of vaccine preparation had been reported earlier [TERSKIKH *et al.*, 1964].

ii) Vaccination. The course of vaccinotherapy included three subconjunctival and subcutaneous injections of vaccine at 7-day intervals. 100 patients with trachoma stage III and 12 patients with trachoma stage I–II were treated. Antirelapse treatment was conducted in 116 patients recovered from trachoma. The efficacy of vaccinotherapy was evaluated according to clinical and microscopical examinations. Scrapings and biopsies were taken repeatedly.

iii) Results. The authors concluded that administration of vaccine to patients with severe trachoma III gave recovery in 70% and improvement in 30% of the cases. However, information on the purity and e.b. content of the vaccine preparations was not available.

f) Vaccination Trials in Gambia

i) The vaccine [SOWA *et al.*, 1969]. The vaccine was prepared from *C. trachomatis* strain MRC-187 isolated from a Gambian child suffering from early trachoma with micropannus. The elementary bodies were purified from infected yolk sacs (at the 6th chick embryo passage level), and the yolk suspensions were treated with 0.5% (w/v) trypsin for 30 min at 37 °C and then subjected to differential centrifugation. Elementary bodies were counted by the method of REEVE and TAVERNE [1962]. On the day of use, the vaccines and control preparations were emulsified in an equal volume of a mixture of 9 parts of mineral oil and 1 part of mannide nono-oleate. The trypsinization step was omitted in the preparation of other vaccines. Each vaccine dose contained $10^{9.0}$ to $10^{9.8}$ elementary bodies.

ii) Results. The mineral-oil adjuvant vaccine prepared from a Gambian strain had a barely significant protection 6 months after immunization. After 2 years, the average severity was increased in the immunized children.

iii) Conclusions. In studies where the vaccine contained less than the critical mass of elementary bodies, an enhancement in the severity of the acquired infection was noted. Improvement of vaccines (purity from yolk sac materials and increased antigenicity) might provide some protection against trachoma. JAWETZ [1967] suggested that elucidation of the aggravated disease following vaccination was needed. The disease is similar to that observed with mycoplasmal and rickettsial vaccines.

iv) Evaluation of the trachoma vaccine. COLLIER [1972, 1973] analyzed the state of vaccination and concluded that 'even when protective or therapeutic effects of vaccination are demonstrable, they are never dramatic in clinical terms, and are rarely so obvious that they are apparent without resort to statistical tests of significance.' COLLIER [1972] also indicated that in the Gambian field trial [SOWA *et al.*, 1969], the incidence of trachoma was similar in immunized and unimmunized groups. The severity of the disease was, on the average, worse in the immunized children. In this analysis, COLLIER also calculated the cost of production of trachoma vaccine prepared in chick embryos or WI-38 human diploid cells. The calculated cost per dose ranges from $ 7.13 (using embryonated eggs for production of elementary bodies) to $ 27.23 (using WI-38 cells for e. b. production), indicating that if one-tenth of the material per dose can be used, the vaccine price could be one-tenth of the estimated cost. In contrast, the cost of tetracycline is $ 0.20 for an oily suspension which can be used for one cycle of treatment per person. In view of the cost of vaccine production and the lack of knowledge of methods to improve vaccination and to prevent side effects (like hypersensitivity), it seems that further research on the purification of trachoma antigens and the method of immunization (local or systemic) is needed to facilitate research on methods for trachoma prevention and control.

IX. Summary and Conclusions

Recent developments in the research on trachoma have led to a clearer understanding of the chlamydial agents, both from their systematic position and their biological properties. The research on trachoma is still in a developmental stage, aiming to resolve the nature of the obligate parasitism of the agents and to devise ways to control the diseases caused by the members of the group.

The development of techniques to isolate the agents of trachoma from a large number of patients opened the way to the classification and characterization of the agents. It is now recognized that the chlamydiae differ from Rickettsiae and are members of a new order Chlamydiales [PAGE, 1966, 1968, 1973]. Studies on the biology of chlamydial agents cultivated *in vitro* led to the demonstration that chlamydial agents can be divided according to their properties into two distinct species: (a) *Chlamydia trachomatis* and (b) *Chlamydia psittaci* [STORZ and PAGE, 1971]. The use of DNA hybridization techniques made possible the demonstration [WEISS, 1971] that *C. trachomatis* and *C. psittaci* are quite remote from each other. This finding could lead to the suggestion that *C. trachomatis* and *C. psittaci* should be put in two separate families within the new order Chlamydiales. The use of immunological techniques demonstrated that *C. trachomatis* agents can be divided into nine distinct antigenic types which are related to each other in a manner that suggests a possible evolutionary trait. WANG and GRAYSTON [1972] and WANG *et al.* [1973] concluded that the lymphogranuloma venereum (LGV) strains might be the earliest strains historically, from which the genital TRIC agents may have been derived. The ocular trachoma strains represent the most recent development of chlamydial strains.

One of the major difficulties encountered in trachoma research was the isolation, in embryonated eggs, of the trachoma agents from specimens obtained from the eyes of trachoma patients [TARIZZO *et al.*, 1968]. The development of a cell culture system (irradiated McCoy cells) sensitive to trachoma agents made possible the direct isolation and characterization of numerous trachoma strains. However, the difficulty of the continuous propagation of trachoma agents in cultured cells has not yet been resolved. The relative ease in the propagation of LGV strains as compared to the difficulties with the continuous propagation of trachoma agents indicated a possible difference in the nature of the two types of agents. The reason for the obligate parasitism of *C. trachomatis* is not yet understood. Purification of the trachoma infectious elementary bodies (e.b.) led to the demonstration that the e.b. contain DNA-dependent RNA polymerase molecules which are responsible for the synthesis of RNA within the developing e.b. It is possible to assume that the activation of this trachoma enzyme, an essential step in the developmental cycle, is dependent on host cell processes [BECKER, 1972a, b]. It was also demonstrated [BECKER and ASHER, 1972a] that mitochondrial functions are essential for the development of the trachoma agent. Further studies are needed for the elucidation of the nature of the obligate parasitism of the trachoma agent.

The purification of trachoma e.b. made possible the analysis of the agent's macromolecules. It was found that the e.b. is a prokaryotic cell with a DNA genome (660 × 10^6 daltons molecular weight), ribosomal subunits [SAROV and BECKER, 1968, 1969], numerous proteins [BECKER *et al.*, 1971] and seven distinct antigenic components [KATZENELSON and BERNKOPF, 1967]. The group-specific antigen which has a hemagglutinin activity [ZAKAY-RONES *et al.*, 1968] has been extracted, and its carbohydrate moiety was identified as 2-keto-3 deoxyoctanoic acid [DHIR *et al.*, 1972]. Further characterization of the group- and species-specific antigens is needed to characterize the antigenic composition of *C. trachomatis*.

Electron microscopy of *C. trachomatis*-infected cells revealed the various developmental stages of the agent. Studies by KRAMER and GORDON [1971] and BECKER [unpublished] demonstrated that the elementary bodies are formed from larger bodies (initial or secondary bodies) by a process which resembles binary fission. The exact mechanism by which the latter structures are formed during the early developmental stages is not yet known. Molecular studies demonstrated that, prior to the formation of the e.b., a high rate of RNA and protein synthesis was noted in the trachoma inclusions, but only a low rate of DNA synthesis was detected. The formation of the elementary bodies is associated with a burst in the synthesis of trachoma DNA [BECKER *et al.*, 1971; GUTTER and BECKER, 1972]. These results indicated that e.b. are formed by a process resembling binary fission, and the trachoma DNA genomes are duplicated during this process in order to transfer a complete genome to each of the daughter cells. The low level of DNA synthesis during the initial phase, prior to the formation of e.b., might indicate that some duplication of the parental DNA genome was necessary in order to enable the formation of initial bodies. The mechanisms involved in the morphogenesis of trachoma agent are still to be studied. It is possible that if temperature-sensitive mutants of *C. trachomatis* could be obtained, the studies on the molecular processes during the development of *C. trachomatis* would be enhanced.

The analysis of the developing chlamydia demonstrated that the synthesis of RNA and of proteins resembles that of prokaryotic cells. This property of *C. trachomatis* made possible the selective inhibition of the host cell processes and the study of the parasite's metabolism [BECKER and ASHER, 1972b]. It is possible to assume that further studies might lead to a better understanding of the synthesis of trachoma membranes and cell wall components as well as the mechanisms which control trachoma development.

The chemotherapy of trachoma infections is based on the prokaryotic nature of *C. trachomatis*. Most of the antibacterial antibiotics, as well as sulfa drugs, inhibit trachoma development. However, not all the antitrachoma drugs or antibiotics are also effective in the treatment of trachoma infections in the human eye. Long-acting sulfonamides were suggested for effective treatment of trachoma patients [BIETTI *et al.*, 1964]. The most effective antibiotics now in use are the tetracyclines [TARIZZO and NATAF, 1970]. Further studies on new antibiotics might lead to the development of more effective and potent antibiotics which will be useful in the treatment of trachoma patients in endemic regions. One such possibility was indicated by the study of rifampicin [BECKER and ZAKAY-RONES, 1969]. This antibiotic irreversibly inhibits the trachoma agent in experimental systems, but the value of the antibiotic for treatment of trachoma patients is still to be explored. Another approach to trachoma therapy might be the use of interferon inducers or interferon, which was found to inhibit trachoma development in cultured cells [HANNA *et al.*, 1966, 1967]. The mechanism by which interferon inhibits trachoma development is not yet known, but the finding that interferon does block trachoma development suggests that further studies on this problem are necessary.

The control of trachoma infections by immunization was the goal of a large number of studies. It was hoped, shortly after the successful isolation of trachoma agents, that the preparation of trachoma vaccine would be readily achieved and that vaccination of trachoma patients as well as uninfected humans in endemic areas would reduce the severity and the distribution of the disease. It was found, however, that immunization resulted in a lack of protection against trachoma infections and in an increased sensitization. The studies on trachoma agents during the last decade revealed that many types of trachoma strains exist in different parts of the world and that small doses of unpurified elementary bodies (less than 10^9 e. b. per dose) are insufficient for immunization and result in a more severe infection [GRAYSTON *et al.*, 1971]. The development of techniques for the purification of trachoma e. b. and the extraction of the antigens which are important in the development of immunization against trachoma might lead to the production of potent antitrachoma vaccines.

Immunological studies on antitrachoma antibodies directed attention to the local antibodies present in the excretions of trachoma-infected human eyes [BERNKOPF *et al.*, 1966b]. Local immunization of the eyes, as well as the immunological responses to systemic immunization, are still in a study phase. Further research is needed to study the properties of neutralizing antitrachoma antibodies.

It is hoped that studies during the next decade will help to resolve the mechanisms of trachoma parasitism, the molecular processes of its development, the role of trachoma antigens in immunity and the control of this world-wide disease.

X. References

ADESNIK, M. and LEVINTHAL, C.: Synthesis and maturation of ribosomal RNA in *Escherichia coli.* J. molec. Biol. *46:* 281–303 (1969).

ALEXANDER, E. R.; WANG, S. P., and GRAYSTON, J. T.: Further classification of TRIC agents from ocular trachoma and other sources by the mouse toxicity prevention test. Amer. J. Ophthal. *63:* 1469–1478 (1967).

BARRON, A. L. and COLLINS, A. R.: Studies on trachoma agent by double diffusion gel precipitation. Amer. J. Ophthal. *63:* 1487–1491 (1967).

BARRON, A. L.; MOUNT, D. T.; CORNELL, D. S., and BRODY, H.: Growth of chlamydial agents in organ cultures of primate ocular tissue; in NICHOLS Trachoma and related disorders caused by chlamydial agents. Excerpta med. Int. Congr. Series No. 223, pp. 71–78 (1971).

BARRON, A. L.; ZAKAY-RONES, Z., and BERNKOPF, H.: Hemagglutination of chicken erythrocytes by the agent of psittacosis. Proc. Soc. exp. Biol. Med. *119:* 377–381 (1965).

BARWELL, C. F.; DUNLOP, E., and RACE, J. W.: Results of complement-fixation and intradermal tests for Bedsoniae in genital infection, disease of the eye and Reiter's disease. Amer. J. Ophthal. *63:* 1527–1534 (1967).

BECKER, Y.: Antitrachoma activity of rifamycin B and 8-O-acetylrifamycin S. Nature, Lond. *231:* 115–116 (1971 a).

BECKER, Y.: Cure and eradication of trachoma agent by the antibiotic rifamycin. 21st Conc. Ophthalmology, Mexico City 1970. Excerpta med. Int. Congr. Series No. 222, pp. 1921–1926 (1971 b).

BECKER, Y.: Rifampicin – an antitrachoma antibiotic. Israel J. med. Sci. *8:* 1110–1113 (1972a).

BECKER, Y.: The molecular biology of trachoma agent. Israel J. med. Sci. *8:* 1134–1137 (1972b).

BECKER, Y. and ASHER, Y.: Obligate parasitism of trachoma agent: lack of trachoma development in ethidium bromide-treated cells. Antimicrobial Agents Chemother. *1:* 171–173 (1972a).

BECKER, Y. and ASHER, Y.: Synthesis of trachoma agent proteins in emetine treated cells. J. Bact. *109:* 966–970 (1972b).

BECKER, Y.; ASHER, Y.; HIMMEL, N., and ZAKAY-RONES, Z.: Antitrachoma activity of rifampicin and rifamycin SV derivatives. Nature, Lond. *225:* 454–455 (1970).

BECKER, Y.; ASHER, Y.; HIMMEL, N.; ZAKAY-RONES, Z., and MAYTHAR, B.: Rifampicin inhibition of trachoma agent *in vivo.* Nature, Lond. *224:* 33–34 (1969a).

BECKER, Y.; HOCHBERG, E., and ZAKAY-RONES, Z.: Interaction of trachoma elementary bodies with host cells. Israel J. med. Sci. *5:* 121–124 (1969b).

BECKER, Y.; LOKER, H.; SAROV, I.; ASHER, Y.; GUTTER, B., and ZAKAY-RONES, Z.:

Studies on the molecular biology of trachoma agent; in NICHOLS Trachoma and related disorders caused by chlamydial agents. Excerpta med. Int. Congr. Series No. 223, pp. 13–26 (1971).

BECKER, Y.; MASHIAH, P., and BERNKOPF, H.: Biochemical changes in FL cell-cultures infected with a trachoma agent. Nature, Lond. *193:* 271–272 (1962).

BECKER, Y.; MASHIAH, P., and BERNKOPF, H.: Electron microscope observations on the growth cycle of trachoma agent in FL cell cultures. Bull. Res. Council Israel *10E:* 160–177 (1963).

BECKER, Y. and SAROV, I.: Electron microscopy of vaccinia virus DNA. J. molec. Biol. *34:* 655–660 (1968).

BECKER, Y. and ZAKAY-RONES, Z.: Rifampicin – a new antitrachoma drug. Nature, Lond. *222:* 851–853 (1969).

BEDSON, S. P. and BLAND, J. O. W.: A morphological study of psittacosis virus, with the description of a developmental cycle. Brit. J. exp. Path. *13:* 461–466 (1932).

BELL, S. D., Jr. and MCCOMB, D. E.: Differentiation of trachoma Bedsoniae *in vitro*. Proc. Soc. exp. Biol. Med. *124:* 34–39 (1967).

BELL, S. D., Jr. and THEOBALD, B.: Differentiation of trachoma strains on the basis of immunization against toxic death of mice. Ann. N.Y. Acad. Sci. *98:* 337–346 (1962).

BERNKOPF, H.: The susceptibility of white mice to a strain of trachoma virus and their use in neutralization tests. Bull. Res. Council Israel *8E:* 25–29 (1959).

BERNKOPF, H.: Trachoma virus – recent developments. Progr. med. Virol., vol. 4, pp. 119–156 (Karger, Basel 1962).

BERNKOPF, H.: A plaque test for TRIC agents. Amer. J. Ophthal. *63:* 1206–1207 (1967).

BERNKOPF, H. and MASHIAH, P.: The growth cycle of a trachoma agent in FL cell cultures. J. Immunol. *88:* 570–571 (1962).

BERNKOPF, H.; MASHIAH, P., and BECKER, Y.: Correlation between morphological and biochemical changes and the appearance of infectivity in FL cell cultures infected with trachoma agent. Ann. N.Y. Acad. Sci. *98:* 62–81 (1962a).

BERNKOPF, H.; MASHIAH, P., and BECKER, Y.: Susceptibility of a trachoma agent grown in FL cell cultures to the action of antibiotics and a sulfa drug. Proc. Soc. exp. Biol. Med. *111:* 61–67 (1962b).

BERNKOPF, H.; MASHIAH, P., and MAYTHAR, B.: Cultivation of a strain of trachoma virus in the FL line of human amnion cells. Bull. Res. Council Israel *8E:* 121–127 (1960).

BERNKOPF, H. and NISHMI, M.: Assay of the antigenic properties of trachoma agent preparations in guinea pigs. Amer. J. Ophthal. *63:* 1479–1482 (1967).

BERNKOPF, H.; NISHMI, M.; MAYTHAR, B., and FEITELBERG, I.: Trachoma infection in a human volunteer produced by egg-cultured virus. Arch. Ophthal., Chicago *62:* 33–34 (1959).

BERNKOPF, H.; ORFILA, J., and BABUDIERI, B.: Review on the serology and immunology of trachoma. Rev. int. Trach. *43:* 8–26 (1966a).

BERNKOPF, H.; ORFILA, J., and MAYTHAR, B.: Fluorescent antibodies in the fluid of the conjunctival sac of trachoma patients. Nature, Lond. *209:* 725–726 (1966b).

BERNKOPF, H.; TREU, G., and MAYTHAR, B.: Human infection experiments with three cell-cultured trachoma agents. Arch. Ophthal., Chicago *71:* 693–700 (1964).

BIETTI, G. B.; BUOGO, A. N.; GHIONE, M.; GUERRA, P.; SOLDATI, M., and VOZZA, R.:

Studies on an antitrachoma vaccine: evaluation of its activity on the basis of laboratory and clinical experiments. Proc. 4th Afro-Asian Congr. Ophthalmology, pp. 1–14 (1968).

Bietti, G. B.; Buogo, A.; Ghione, M., and Milano, C.: Skin reactions with several trachoma antigens. Amer. J. Ophthal. *63:* 1513–1520 (1967a).

Bietti, G. B.; Pannarale, C., and Milano, C.: Further contributions to the intermittent therapy of trachoma with new long-acting sulfonamides. Amer. J. Ophthal *63:* 1569–1573 (1967b).

Bietti, G. B.; Guerra, P.; Felici, A., and Vozza, R.: Role of trachoma vaccine in prevention and treatment of the experimental and natural disease. Orient. A. Ophthal. *1963:* 76–92.

Bietti, G. B.; Guerra, P.; Felici, A., and Vozza, R.: Results of antitrachoma vaccination trials in East Africa. J. all-India ophthal. Soc. *12:* 59–64 (1964).

Bietti, G. B.; Guerra, P.; Felici, A., and Vozza, R.: Results of antitrachoma vaccination trials in East Africa. Acta Soc. ophthal. jap. *69:* 34–53 (1965).

Bietti, G. B.; Guerra, P.; Vozza, R.; Felici, A.; Ghione, M.; Buogo, A.; Lolli, B.; Salomons, H., and Kebreth, Y.: Results of large-scale vaccination against trachoma. Amer. J. Ophthal. *61:* 1010–1029 (1966).

Bietti, G. B. et Vozza, R.: Le trachome. Revue générale des travaux parus dans la période de 1951 à 1960. Progr. Ophthal., vol. *13*, pp. 132–261 (Karger, Basel 1963).

Bietti, G. B. and Werner, G. H.: Trachoma: prevention and treatment, p. 227 (Thomas, Springfield 1967).

Blyth, W. A.: Studies on TRIC organisms in tissues of normal and immune guinea pigs. Amer. J. Ophthal. *63:* 1153–1161 (1967).

Blyth, W. A.; Taverne, J., and Garret, A. J.: Trachoma inclusions separated from cells; in Nichols Trachoma and related disorders caused by chlamydial agents. Excerpta Medica International Congress Series No. 223, pp. 79–87 (1971).

Bode, H. R. and Morowitz, H. J.: Size and structure of the *Mycoplasma hominis* H39 chromosome. J. molec. Biol. *23:* 191–199 (1967).

Cairns, J.: The chromosome of *Escherichia coli.* Cold Spr. Harb. Symp. quant. Biol. *28:* 43–46 (1963).

Casazza, A. M.; Intini, C.; Verini, M. A., and Ghione, M.: Preliminary studies on mouse macrophage cultures infected with trachoma agents. Experientia *25:* 327–329 (1969).

Collier, L. H.: Observations of trachoma virus isolated in embryonated eggs. Rev. int. Trach. *36:* 57–65 (1959a).

Collier, L. H.: Recent advances in the virology of trachoma, inclusion conjunctivitis and allied diseases. Brit. med. Bull. *15:* 231–234 (1959b).

Collier, L. H.: Growth characteristics of inclusion blennorrhea virus in cell cultures. Ann. N.Y. Acad. Sci. *98:* 42–49 (1962).

Collier, L. H.: in Nichols Trachoma and related disorders caused by chlamydial agents. Excerpta med. Int. Congr. Series No. 223, p. 363 (1971).

Collier, L. H.: Some aspects of trachoma control and provisional estimates of the cost of vaccine production. Israel J. med. Sci. *8:* 1114–1123 (1972).

Collier, L. H.: Life at a border. A review of the work of the MRC trachoma unit. Ann. Rep. Lister Inst., pp. 1–26 (1973).

Collier, L. H.; Blyth, W. A.; Larin, N. M., and Treharne, J.: Immunogenicity of experimental trachoma vaccines in baboons. III. Experiments with inactivated vaccines. J. Hyg. *65:* 97–107 (1967).

Collier, L. H.; Duke-Elder, S., and Jones, B. R.: Experimental trachoma produced by cultured virus. Brit. J. Ophthal. *42:* 705–720 (1958).

Collier, L. H. and Smith, A.: Dissemination and immunogenicity of live TRIC agent in baboons after parenteral injection. Amer. J. Ophthal. *63:* 1589–1602 (1967).

Collier, L. H. and Sowa, J.: Isolation of trachoma virus in embryonated eggs. Lancet *i:* 993–996 (1958).

Collier, L. H.; Sowa, J., and Sowa, S.: The serum and conjunctival antibody response to trachoma in Gambian children. J. Hyg. *70:* 727–740 (1972).

Collins, A. R. and Barron, A. L.: Demonstration of group and species-specific antigens of chlamydial agents by gel diffusion. J. infect. Dis. *121:* 1–8 (1970).

Colon, J. I.: Enzymes for formation of citrovorum factor in members of the psittacosis group of microorganisms. J. Bact. *79:* 741–746 (1960).

Colon, J. I. and Moulder, J. W.: Folic acid in purified preparations of members of the psittacosis group of micro-organisms. J. infect. Dis. *103:* 109–119 (1958).

Cox, H. R.: Viral and rickettsial toxins. Annu. Rev. Microbiol. *7:* 197–218 (1953).

Darougar, S. and Jones, B. R.: Conjunctival swabbing for the isolation of TRIC agent (chlamydia). Brit. J. Ophthal. *55:* 585–590 (1971).

Darougar, S.; Kinnison, J. R., and Jones, B. R.: Simplified irradiated McCoy cell culture for isolation of *Chlamydiae*; in Nichols Trachoma and related disorders caused by chlamydial agents. Excerpta med. Int. Congr. Series No. 223, pp. 63–70 (1971a).

Darougar, S.; Dwyer, R. St. C.; Treharne, J. D.; Harper, I. A.; Garland, J. A., and Jones, B. R.: A comparison of laboratory methods of diagnosis of chlamydial infection; in Nichols Trachoma and related disorders caused by chlamydial agents. Excerpta med. Int. Congr. Series No. 223, pp. 445–460 (1971b).

Dawson, C. R.; Ostler, H. B.; Hanna, L.; Hoshiwara, I., and Jawetz, E.: Tetracyclines in the treatment of chronic trachoma in American Indians. J. infect. Dis. *124:* 255–263 (1971).

Dawson, C. R. and Schachter, J.: TRIC agent infections of the eye and the genital tract. Amer. J. Ophthal. *63:* 1288–1298 (1967).

Dhir, S. P.; Agarwal, L. P.; Detels, R.; Wang, S. P., and Grayston, J. T.: Field trial of two bivalent trachoma vaccines in children of Punjab Indian villages. Amer. J. Ophthal. *63:* 1639–1644 (1967).

Dhir, S. P.; Hakomori, S.; Kenny, G. E., and Grayston, J. T.: Immunochemical studies on chlamydial group antigen. (Presence of a 2-keto-3 deoxycarbohydrate as immunodominant group.) J. Immunol. *109:* 116–122 (1972).

Dunlop, E. M. C.; Hare, M. J.; Darougar, S., and Jones, B. R.: Chlamydial infection of the urethra in men presenting because of 'non-specific' urethritis; in Nichols Trachoma and related disorders caused by chlamydial agents. Excerpta med. Int. Congr. Series No. 223, pp. 494–500 (1971a).

Dunlop, E. M. C.; Hare, M. J.; Darougar, S., and Jones, B. R.: Chlamydial isolates from the rectum in association with chlamydial infection of the eye or genital tract. II. Clinical aspects; in Nichols Trachoma and related disorders caused by chlamydial agents. Excerpta med. Int. Congr. Series No. 223, pp. 507–512 (1971b).

ERLANDSON, R. A. and ALLEN, E. G.: The ultrastructure of meningopneumonitis. Virology *22:* 410–418 (1964).

EVANS, A.: The development of TRIC organisms in cell cultures during multiple infection. J. Hyg. *70:* 39–48 (1972).

FAN, V. S. C. and JENKIN, H. M.: Glycogen metabolism in chlamydia infected HeLa cells. J. Bact. *104:* 608–609 (1970).

FINDLAY, G. M.; MACKENZIE, R. D., and MACCALLUM, F. O.: A morphological study of the virus of lymphogranuloma inguinale (climatic bubo). Trans. roy. Soc. trop. Med. Hyg. *32:* 183–188 (1938).

FOY, H. M.; WANG, S. P.; KENNY, G. E.; JOHNSON, W. L., and GRAYSTON, J. T.: Isolation of TRIC agents and mycoplasma from the cervix of pregnant women. Amer. J. Ophthal. *63:* 1053–1056 (1967).

FRIIS, R. R.: Interaction of L cells and *Chlamydia psittaci:* entry of the parasite and host response to its development. J. Bact. *110:* 706–721 (1972).

FURNESS, G. and FRASER, E. F.: One step growth curves for inclusion blennorrhea virus in HeLa cell monolayers. J. gen. Microbiol. *27:* 299–304 (1962).

FURNESS, G.; GRAHAM, D. M., and REEVE, P.: The titration of trachoma and inclusion blennorrhea viruses in cell cultures. J. gen. Microbiol. *23:* 613–619 (1960a).

FURNESS, G.; GRAHAM, D. M.; REEVE, P., and COLLIER, L. H.: The growth of trachoma and inclusion blennorrhea viruses in cell culture. Rev. int. Trach. *37:* 574–584 (1960b).

FURNESS, G.; HENDERSON, W. G.; CSONKA, G. W., and FRASER, E. F.: A study by fluorescence microscopy of the replication of inclusion blennorrhea virus in HeLa cell monolayers. J. gen. Microbiol. *28:* 571–578 (1962).

GEAR, J. H. S.; CUTHBERTSON, E., and RYAN, J.: Trachoma: laboratory studies of trachoma and related infections in South Africa. Amer. J. Ophthal. *63:* 1310–1312 (1967).

GEAR, J. H. S.; GORDON, F. B.; JONES, B. R., and BELL, S. D.: Nomenclature of isolates of virus from trachoma and inclusion blennorrhea. Nature, Lond. *197:* 26 (1963).

GILKES, M. J.; SMITH, C. H., and SOWA, J.: Trachoma inclusions and penicillin. Brit. J. Ophthalmol. *42:* 478–482 (1958).

GORDON, F. B.; DRESSLER, H. R., and QUAN, A. L.: Relative sensitivity of cell culture and yolk sac for detection of TRIC infection. Amer. J. Ophthal *63:* 1044–1048 (1967).

GORDON, F. B.; HARPER, I. A.; QUAN, A. L.; TREHARNE, J. D.; DWYER, R. ST. C., and GARLAND, J. A.: Detection of chlamydia (Bedsonia) in certain infections of man. 1. Laboratory procedures: comparison of yolk-sac and cell culture for detection and isolation. J. infect. Dis. *120:* 451–462 (1969).

GORDON, F. B.; MAGRUDER, G. B.; QUAN, A. L., and ARM, H. G.: Cell cultures for detection of trachoma virus from experimental simian infections. Proc. Soc. exp. Biol. Med. *112:* 236–242 (1963).

GORDON, F. B.; NICHOLS, R. L., and QUAN, A. L.: Immunotyping of *Chlamydia trachomatis* with fluorescent antibody: retention of immunospecificity in cell culture passage, and typing with infected cell monolayers; in NICHOLS Trachoma and related disorders caused by chlamydial agents. Excerpta med. Int. Congr. Series No. 223, pp. 358–362 (1971).

GORDON, F. B. and QUAN, A. L.: Occurrence of glycogen in inclusions of the psittacosis-lymphogranuloma venereum-trachoma agents. J. infect. Dis *115:* 186–196 (1965a).

GORDON, F. B. and QUAN, A. L.: Isolation of the trachoma agent in cell culture. Proc. Soc. exp. Biol. Med. *118:* 354–359 (1965b).

GORDON, F. B. and QUAN, A. L.: Isolation of *Chlamydia trachomatis* from the human genital tract by cell culture: a summary; in NICHOLS Trachoma and related disorders caused by chlamydial agents. Excerpta med. Int. Congr. Series No. 223, pp. 476–484 (1971).

GORDON, F. B.; QUAN, A. L., and TRIMMER, R. W.: Morphologic observations on trachoma virus in cell cultures. Science *131:* 733–734 (1960).

GRAHAM, D. M.: Growth and immunogenicity of TRIC agents in mice. Amer. J. Ophthal. *63:* 1173–1190 (1967).

GRAHAM, D. M. and LAYTON, J. E.: The induction of chlamydia group antibody in rabbits inoculated with trachoma agents and demonstration of strain-specific neutralizing antibody in sera; in NICHOLS Trachoma and related disorders caused by chlamydial agents. Excerpta med. Int. Congr. Series No. 223, pp. 145–157 (1971).

GRAYSTON, J. T.: Immunization against trachoma. 1st Int. Conf. Vaccines against Viral and Rickettsial Diseases of Man. PAHO Scientific Publication No. 147, p. 546 (1967).

GRAYSTON, J. T.: Summary of conference; in NICHOLS Trachoma and related disorders caused by chlamydial agents. Excerpta med. Int. Congr. Series No. 223, pp. 568–572 (1971).

GRAYSTON, J. T.; KIM, K. S. W.; ALEXANDER, E. R., and WANG, S. P.: Protective studies in monkeys with trivalent and monovalent trachoma vaccines; in NICHOLS Trachoma and related disorders caused by chlamydial agents. Excerpta med. Int. Congr. Series No. 223, pp. 377–385 (1971).

GRAYSTON, J. T.; WANG, S. P., and JOHNSTON, P. B.: Etiologic studies of trachoma on Taiwan. Proc. Soc. exp. Biol. Med. *103:* 596–599 (1960).

GRAYSTON, J. T.; WOOLRIDGE, R. L., and WANG, S. P.: Trachoma vaccine studies on Taiwan. Ann. N.Y. Acad. Sci. *98:* 352–367 (1962).

GUERRA, P.; AOKI, K., and BUOGO, A.: The treatment of trachoma with vaccine and long acting sulfonamide combinations compared with treatment with vaccine and sulfonamide only; in PUIG and SOLANES 21st Conc. Ophthalmology, Mexico City 1970. Excerpta med. Int. Congr. Series No. 222, pp. 1876–1880 (1971).

GUERRA, P.; BUOGO, B. D.; MARUBINI, E., and GHIONE, M.: Analysis of clinical and laboratory data of an experiment with trachoma vaccine in Ethiopia. Amer. J. Ophthal *63:* 1631–1638 (1967).

GUPTA, V. C.; PARTHASARATHY, N. R., and GUPTA, C. K.: Study of broad spectrum antibiotic Kajal in mass control of trachoma. Amer. J. Ophthal *65:* 778–781 (1968).

GUTTER, B.; ASHER, Y.; COHEN, Y., and BECKER, Y.: Studies on the developmental cycle of *C. trachomatis*. Isolation and characterization of the initial bodies. J. Bact. *115:* 691–702 (1973).

GUTTER, B. and BECKER, Y.: Synthesis and maturation of ribosomal RNA during the developmental cycle of trachoma agent, a prokaryotic obligate parasite of eukaryocytes. J. molec. Biol. *66:* 239–253 (1972).

HALBERSTAEDTER, L. and VON PROWAZEK, S.: Zur Aetiologie des Trachoms. Dtsch. med. Wschr. *33:* 1285–1287 (1907).

HANNA, L.: Isolation of trachoma and inclusion conjunctivitis viruses in the United States. Ann. N.Y. Acad. Sci. *98:* 24–30 (1962).

HANNA, L.: Glossary. Amer. J. Ophthal. *63:* 1657 (1967).

HANNA, L.; JAWETZ, E.; NABLI, B.; HOSHIWARA, I.; OSTLER, B., and DAWSON, C.: Titration and typing of serum antibodies in TRIC infections by immunofluorescence. J. Immunol. *108:* 102–107 (1972).

HANNA, L.; JAWETZ, E.; THYGESON, P., and DAWSON, C.: Trachoma viruses isolated in United States. I. Growth in embryonated eggs. Proc. Soc. exp. Biol. Med. *104:* 142–145 (1960).

HANNA, L.; MERIGAN, T. C., and JAWETZ, E.: Inhibition of TRIC agents by virus induced interferon. Proc. Soc. exp. Biol. Med. *122:* 417–421 (1966).

HANNA, L.; MERIGAN, T. C., and JAWETZ, E.: Effect of interferon on TRIC agents and induction of interferon by TRIC agents. Amer. J. Ophthal *63:* 1115–1119 (1967).

HANNA, L.; THYGESON, P., and JAWETZ, E.: Elementary-body virus isolated from clinical trachoma in California. Science *130:* 1339–1340 (1959).

HATHAWAY, A. and PETERS J. H.: Characterization of antibodies to trachoma in human eye secretions; in NICHOLS Trachoma and related disorders caused by chlamydial agents. Excerpta med. Int. Congr. Series No. 223, pp. 260–268 (1971).

HIGASHI, N.: The mode of reproduction of the psittacosis-lymphogranuloma-trachoma (PLT) group viruses. Int. Rev. exp. Path. *3:* 35–64 (1964).

HIGASHI, N.; TAMURA, A., and IWANAGA, M.: Developmental cycle and reproductive mechanism of the meningopneumonitis virus in strain L cells. Ann. N.Y. Acad. Sci. *98:* 100–121 (1962).

HOLT, S.; PEDERSEN, A. H. B.; WANG, S. P.; KENNY, G. E.; FOY, H. M., and GRAYSTON, J. T.: Isolation of TRIC agents and mycoplasma from the genito-urinary tracts of patients of a venereal disease clinic. Amer. J. Ophthal. *63:* 1057–1064 (1967).

HOSHIWARA, I.; OSTER, B.; HANNA, L.; CIGNETTI, F.; COLEMAN, V. R., and JAWETZ, E.: Doxycycline treatment of chronic trachoma. J. amer. med. Ass. *224:* 220–223 (1973).

HURST, E. W. and REEVE, P.: Transmission of viruses of trachoma, inclusion blennorrhea and lymphogranuloma to mice. Nature, Lond. *186:* 336 (1960).

ISA, A. M.: The antibody response to chlamydial agents. I. Studies in the monkey; in NICHOLS Trachoma and related disorders caused by chlamydial agents. Excerpta med. Int. Congr. Series No. 223, pp. 196–205 (1971).

JAWETZ, E.: Seasonal insusceptibility of embryonated eggs to viruses of trachoma and inclusion conjunctivitis. Ann. N.Y. Acad. Sci. *98:* 31–37 (1962a).

JAWETZ, E.: Discussion. Ann. N.Y. Acad. Sci. *98:* 278–280 (1962b).

JAWETZ, E.: Agents of trachoma and inclusion conjunctivitis. Annu. Rev. Microbiol. *18:* 301–334 (1964).

JAWETZ, E.: Discussion of papers 67–73. Amer. J. Ophthal. *63:* 1654–1655 (1967).

JAWETZ, E.: Chemotherapy of chlamydial infections. Adv. Pharmacol. Chemother. *7:* 253–282 (1969).

JAWETZ, E.: Discussion; in NICHOLS Trachoma and related disorders caused by chlamydial agents. Excerpta med. Int. Congr. Series No. 223, pp. 562–563 (1971).

JAWETZ, E.; DAWSON, C. R.; SCHACHTER, J.; JUCHAU, V.; NABLI, B., and HANNA, L.: Immunoglobulin nature of antibodies in chlamydial infections; in NICHOLS Trachoma and related disorders caused by chlamydial agents. Excerpta med. Int. Congr. Series No. 223, pp. 233–242 (1971).

JENKIN, H. M.: Preparation and properties of cell walls of the agent of meningopneumonitis. J. Bact. *80:* 639–649 (1960).

JENKIN, H. M.: The continuous passage of agents of trachoma in cell culture. I. Characteristics of TW-3 and Bour strains of trachoma cultivated in serial passage in HeLa 229 cells. J. infect. Dis. *116:* 390–399 (1966).

JENKIN, H. M.: Comparative lipid composition of psittacosis and trachoma agents. Amer. J. Ophthal *63:* 1087–1098 (1967).

JENKIN, H. M. and FAN, V. S. C.: Contrast of glycogenesis of *Chlamydia trachomatis* and *Chlamydia psittaci* strains in HeLa cells; in NICHOLS Trachoma and related disorders caused by chlamydial agents. Excerpta med. Int. Congr. Series No. 223, pp. 52–59 (1971).

JENKIN, H. M. and LU, Y. K.: Induction of an interferon-like effect in HeLa 229 cells by a trachoma agent (Bour). Bact. Proc. *1966:* 121.

JENKIN, H. M. and LU, Y. K.: Induction of interferon by the Bour strain of trachoma in HeLa 229 cells. Amer. J. Ophthal *63:* 1110–1115 (1967).

JOHNSTON, P. B.; GRAYSTON, J. T., and CHEN, P. C.: Development of sulfa resistant variant of trachoma virus. Ann. N.Y. Acad. Sci. *98:* 283 (1962).

JONES, B. R.: Ocular syndromes of TRIC virus infection and their possible genital significance. Brit. J. vener. Dis. *40:* 3 (1964).

JONES, B. R.: Advances and prospects in the study of certain diseases due to infections by subgroup A chlamydia. Brit. J. vener. Dis. *48:* 13–17 (1972).

JONES, B. R.; AL-HUSSAINI, M. K., and DUNLOP, E. M. C.: Infection of the eye and genital tract by TRIC agent. III. Ocular syndromes associated with infection of the genital tract by TRIC agent. Rev. int. Trach. *42:* 27–43 (1965).

JONES, B. R. and COLLIER, L. H.: Inoculation of man with inclusion blennorrhea virus. Ann. N.Y. Acad. Sci. *98:* 212–226 (1962).

JONES, B. R.; COLLIER, L. H., and SMITH, C. H.: Isolation of virus from inclusion blennorrhea. Lancet *i:* 902–905 (1959).

KASSIRA, E. N.: Delayed-type hypersensitivity for differentiation of chlamydial agents; in NICHOLS Trachoma and related disorders caused by chlamydial agents. Excerpta med. Int. Congr. Series No. 223, pp. 177–184 (1971).

KATZENELSON, E. and BERNKOPF, H.: Serologic differentiation of trachoma strains and other agents of the psittacosis-lymphogranuloma venereum-trachoma group with the aid of the direct fluorescent antibody method. J. Immunol. *94:* 467–474 (1965).

KATZENELSON, E. and BERNKOPF, H.: Studies of PLT agents with the aid of agar immune diffusion technique. Amer. J. Ophthal. *63:* 1483–1487 (1967).

KAZAR, J.; GILLMORE, J. D., and GORDON, F. B.: Effect of interferon and interferon inducers on infections with a nonviral intracellular microorganism, *Chlamydia trachomatis*. Infect. Immun. *3:* 825–832 (1971).

KINGSBURY, D. T.: Estimate of the genome size of various microorganisms. J. Bact. *98:* 1400–1401 (1969).

KINGSBURY, D. T. and WEISS, E.: Lack of deoxyribonucleic acid homology between species of the genus chlamydia. J. Bact. *96:* 1421–1423 (1968).

KRAMER, M. J. and GORDON, F. B.: Ultrastructural analysis of the effects of penicillin and chlortetracycline on the development of a genital tract *Chlamydia*. Infect. Immun. *3:* 333–341 (1971).

Kuo, C. C.; Kenny, G. E., and Wang, S. P.: Trachoma and psittacosis antigens in agar gel double immunodiffusion; in Nichols Trachoma and related disorders caused by chlamydial agents. Excerpta med. Int. Congr. Series No. 223, pp. 113–123 (1971a).

Kuo, C. C.; Wang, S. P., and Grayston, J. T.: Studies on delayed hypersensitivity with trachoma organisms. I. Induction of delayed hypersensitivity in guinea pigs and characterization of trachoma allergens; in Nichols Trachoma and related disorders caused by chlamydial agents. Excerpta med. Int. Congr. Series No. 223, pp. 158–167 (1971b).

Kuo, C. C.; Wang, S. P., and Grayston, J. T.: Studies on delayed hypersensitivity with trachoma organisms. II. Demonstration of lymphocyte transformation *in-vitro* by a microtechnique of peripheral blood lymphocyte culture; in Nichols Trachoma and related disorders caused by chlamydial agents. Excerpta med. Int. Congr. Series No. 223, pp. 168–176 (1971c).

Kuo, C. C.; Wang, S. P., and Grayston, J. T.: Differentiation of TRIC and LGV organisms based on enhancement of infectivity by DEAE-dextran in cell culture. J. infect. Dis. *125:* 313–317 (1972a).

Kuo, C. C.; Wang, S. P.; Wentworth, B. B., and Grayston, J. T.: Primary isolation of TRIC organisms in HeLa 229 cells treated with DEAE-dextran. J. infect. Dis. *125:* 665–668 (1972b).

Kurnosova, L. M. and Lenkevich, M. M.: Mode of action of sulfonamides on trachoma virus. Acta Virol., Prague *8:* 350–358 (1964).

Lepine, P.: Recent research on the trachoma virus. Rev. int. Trach. *37:* 562–573 (1960).

Lin, H. S. and Moulder, J. W.: Patterns of response to sulfadiazine, D-cycloserine, and D-alanine in members of the psittacosis group. J. infect. Dis. *116:* 372–376 (1966).

Lindner, K.: Zur Aetiologie der gonokokkenfreien Urethritis. Wien. klin. Wschr. *23:* 283 (1910).

Litwin, J.: The growth cycle of the psittacosis group of microorganisms. J. infect. Dis. *105:* 129–160 (1959).

Litwin, J.; Officer, J. E.; Brown, A., and Moulder, J. W.: A comparative study of the growth cycles of different members of the psittacosis group in different host cells. J. infect. Dis. *109:* 251–279 (1961).

Luria, S. E.: General virology; 1st ed. (Wiley, New York 1953).

Lwoff, A.: The concept of virus. J. gen. Microbiol. *17:* 239–253 (1957).

Lwoff, A. and Tournier, P.: The classification of viruses. Annu. Rev. Microbiol. *20:* 45–74 (1966).

Maizel, J. V.: Acrylamide gel electropherograms by mechanical fractionation: radioactive adenovirus proteins. Science *151:* 988–990 (1966).

McComb, D. E. and Nichols, R. L.: Antibodies to trachoma in eye secretions in Saudi Arab children. Amer. J. Epidem. *90:* 278–284 (1969).

McComb, D. E. and Nichols, R. L.: Antibody type specific to trachoma in eye secretions of Saudi Arab children. Infect. Immun. *2:* 65–68 (1970).

McComb, D. E.; Peters, J. H.; Fraser, C. E. O.; Murray, E. S.; MacDonald, B., and Nichols, R. L.: Resistance to trachoma infection in owl monkeys correlated with antibody status at the outset in an experiment to test the response to topical trachoma antigens; in Nichols Trachoma and related disorders caused by chlamydial agents. Excerpta med. Int. Congr. Series No. 223, pp. 396–406 (1971).

MERIGAN, T. C. and HANNA, L.: Characteristics of interferon induced *in vitro* and *in vivo* by a TRIC agent. Proc. Soc. exp. Biol. Med. *122:* 421–424 (1966).

MEYER, K. F.: Psittacosis-lymphogranuloma group; in RIVERS Viral and rickettsial infections of man, 2nd ed., pp. 441–464 (Lippincott, Philadelphia 1952).

MITSUI, Y.; FUJIMOTO, M., and KAJIMA, M.: Development and morphology of trachoma agent in the yolk sac cell as revealed by electron microscopy. Virology *23:* 30–45 (1964a).

MITSUI, Y.; KITAMURO, T.; ENDO, K., and MATSUMURA, K.: Trachoma and inclusion conjunctivitis agents: adaptation to HeLa cell cultures. Science *145:* 715–716 (1964b).

MITSUI, Y.; HIGAI, H., and KITAMURO, T.: Free toxic substance of trachoma virus. Arch. Ophthal, Chicago *68:* 651–653 (1962a).

MITSUI, Y.; KAJIMA, M.; NISHIMURA, A., and KONISHI, K.: Morphology of trachoma agent in conjunctiva and chick embryo. Ann. N.Y. Acad. Sci. *98:* 131–144 (1962b).

MITSUI, Y.; KITAMURO, T., and FUJIMOTO, M.: Adaptation of TRIC agents to tissue culture and characteristics of tissue culture adapted variants. Amer. J. Ophthal. *63:* 1191–1205 (1967).

MITSUI, Y.; KONISHI, K.; KINOUCHI, T., and KAJIMA, M.: Treatment of trachoma by intramuscular injection of a repository sulfonamide. Amer. J. Ophthal. *55:* 782–787 (1963).

MITSUI, Y.; KONISHI, K., and NISHIMURA, A.: Cultivation of trachoma agent in chick embryo. Acta. Soc. ophthal. jap. *65:* 1110–1113 (1961).

MITSUI, Y.; SUZUKI, A.; HANABUSA, J.; MINODA, R.; OGATA, S.; FUKUSHIMA, S., and MIURA, M.: Structures of the initial bodies of trachoma inclusion as revealed in section by electron microscopy. Virology *6:* 137–149 (1958).

MIZUNO, S.; YAMAZAKI, H.; NITTA, K., and UMEZAWA, H.: Inhibition of DNA dependent RNA polymerase action of *Escherichia coli* by an antimicrobial antibiotic, streptovaricin. Biochim. biophys. Acta *157:* 322–332 (1968).

MOGG, A. E.; COLLIER, L. H., and HARRIS, R. G.: The antibody response to primary and repeated intravenous injections of TRIC agent; in NICHOLS Trachoma and related disorders caused by chlamydial agents. Excerpta med. Int. Congr. Series No. 223, pp. 185–195 (1971).

MORDHORST, C. H.: Isolation of the TRIC agent from 3 cases of neonatal inclusion blennorrhea and from the cervix of one of the mothers. Acta. path. microbiol. scand. *62:* 301–302 (1964).

MORDHORST, C. H.: Isolation of the TRIC agent from eye and urogenital tract of trachoma patients in Denmark. Acta. path. microbiol. scand. *63:* 637–638 (1965a).

MORDHORST, C. H.: TRIC agents isolated in Denmark. 1. Isolation of the TRIC agent from inclusion blennorrhea. Acta. path. microbiol. scand. *64:* 277–285 (1965b).

MORDHORST, C. H.: Studies on oculogenital TRIC agents isolated in Denmark. Amer. J. Ophthal. *63:* 1282–1288 (1967a).

MORDHORST, C. H.: Experimental infections and immunogenicity of TRIC agents in monkeys. Amer. J. Ophthal. *63:* 1603–1615 (1967b).

MORDHORST, C. H.; REINICKE, V., and SCHONNE, E.: *In ovo* inhibition by concentrated chick interferon of the growth of TRIC agents. Amer. J. Ophthal. *63:* 1107–1109 (1967).

MOULDER, J. W.: Structure and chemical composition of isolated particles. Ann. N.Y. Acad. Sci. *98:* 92–99 (1962).

MOULDER, J. W.: The relation of the psittacosis group (chlamydia) to bacteria and viruses. Annu. Rev. Microbiol. *20:* 107–130 (1966).

MOULDER, J. W.: The contribution of model systems to the understanding of infectious diseases. Perspect. Biol. Med. *14:* 486–502 (1971).

MOULDER, J. W.; NOVOSEL, D. L., and OFFICER, J. E.: Inhibition of the growth of agents of the psittacosis group by D-cycloserine and its specific reversal by D-alanine. J. Bact. *85:* 707–711 (1963a).

MOULDER, J. W.; NOVOSEL, D. L., and TRIBBY, I. C.: Diaminopimelic acid decarboxylase of the agent of meningopneumonitis. J. Bact. *85:* 701–706 (1963b).

MURRAY, E. S. and CHARBONNET, L. T.: Experimental conjunctival infection of guinea pigs with guinea pig inclusion conjunctivitis organism; in NICHOLS Trachoma and related disorders caused by chlamydial agents. Excerpta med. Int. Congr. Series No. 223, pp. 369–376 (1971).

MURRAY, E. S.; FRASER, C. E. O.; PETERS, J. H.; MCCOMB, D. E., and NICHOLS, R. L.: The owl monkey as an experimental primate model for conjunctival trachoma infection; in NICHOLS Trachoma and related disorders caused by chlamydial agents. Excerpta med. Int. Congr. Series No. 223, pp. 386–395 (1971).

MURRAY, E. S.; GUERRA, P. A.; ABBOTT, A. G., and MCCOMB, D. E.: Isolation of viruses of trachoma from patients in Ethiopia. Ann. N.Y. Acad. Sci. *98:* 14–23 (1962).

NABLI, B.: The effect of rifampicin on the growth of TRIC agents in embryonated eggs; in NICHOLS Trachoma and related disorders caused by chlamydial agents. Excerpta med. Int. Congr. Series No. 223, pp. 34–39 (1971).

NICHOLS, R. L.; BELL, S. D.; HADDAD, N. A., and BOBB, A. A.: Studies on trachoma. IV. Microbiological observations in a field trial in Saudi Arabia of bivalent trachoma vaccine at three dosage levels. Amer. J. trop. Med. Hyg. *18:* 723–730 (1969).

NICHOLS, R. L.; VON FRITZINGER, K., and MCCOMB, D. E.: Epidemiological data derived from immunotyping of 338 trachoma strains isolated from children in Saudi Arabia; in NICHOLS Trachoma and related disorders caused by chlamydial agents. Excerpta med. Int. Congr. Series No. 223, pp. 337–357 (1971).

NICHOLS, R. L. and MCCOMB, D. E.: Serologic strain differentiation in trachoma. J. exp. Med. *120:* 639–654 (1964).

OH, J. O.; OSTLER, H. B., and SCHACHTER, J.: Effects of interferon inducers on ocular lesions produced by trachoma agent in rabbits; in NICHOLS Trachoma and related disorders caused by chlamydial agents. Excerpta med. Int. Congr. Series No. 223, pp. 533–539 (1971).

OH, J. O.; TARIZZO, M. L., and YONEDA, C.: Growth of trachoma agent in primary cultures of rabbit corneal endothelial cells. J. Bact. *97:* 1502–1503 (1967).

OSSOWSKI, L.; BECKER, Y., and BERNKOPF, H.: Amino acid requirements of trachoma strains and other agents of the PLT group in cell cultures. Israel J. med. Sci. *1:* 186–193 (1965).

OSTLER, H. B.; HANNA, L.; HOSHIWARA, I.; JAWETZ, E., and DAWSON, C. R.: A comparison of tetracycline and doxycycline in chronic trachoma of American Indians; in NICHOLS Trachoma and related disorders caused by chlamydial agents. Excerpta med. Int. Congr. Series No. 223, pp. 540–544 (1971).

OSTLER, H. B.; SCHACHTER, J., and DAWSON, C. R.: Ocular infection of rabbits with a Bedsonia isolated from a patient with Reiter's syndrome. Invest. Ophthal. *9:* 256–262 (1970).

PAGE, L. A.: Revision of the family chlamydiaceae Rake, Rickettsiales, unification of the psittacosis-lymphogranuloma venereum-trachoma group of organisms in the genus chlamydia, Rake and Stearns, 1945. Int. J. syst. Bact. *16:* 223–252 (1966).

PAGE, L. A.: Proposal for the recognition of two species in the genus chlamydia Jones, Rake and Stearns, 1945. Int. J. syst. Bact. *18:* 51–66 (1968).

PAGE, L. A.: Order II chlamydials; in BERGEY, MURRAY and HITCHES Manual of determinative bacteriology, 8th ed. (Williams & Wilkins, Baltimore 1973).

PERKINS, H. R.: Composition of bacterial cell walls in relation to antibiotic action. Adv. Pharmocol. Chemother. *7:* 283–307 (1969).

PERKINS, H. R. and ALLISON, A. C.: Cell-wall constituents of rickettsiae and psittacosis-lymphogranuloma organisms. J. gen. Microbiol. *30:* 469–480 (1963).

PERRET, D. and MANN, I.: Isolation of virus from embryonate eggs inoculated with material from a case of trachoma in Western Australia. Brit. J. Ophthal. *44:* 503–505 (1960).

PETERS, J. H.: Immunogenic and antigenic modification of trachoma Bedsonia. Amer. J. Ophthal. *63:* 1506–1512 (1967).

PETERS, J. H.; MURRAY, E. S.; FRASER, C. E. O.; MCCOMB, D. E.; NICHOLS, R. L.; HATHAWAY, A.; BALDWIN, E.; RADCLIFFE, F.; CHARBONNET, L., and FRITZINGER, K. VON: Development of local and systemic immunity in trachoma of man and animals; in DAYTON, SMALL, CHANOCK, KAUFMAN and TOMASI Secretory immunologic system, p. 341–361 (US Department of Health, Education and Welfare, National Institutes of Health, Washington 1969).

PHILIP, R. N.; HILL, D. A.; GREAVES, A. B.; GORDON, F. B.; QUAN, A. L.; GERLOFF, R. K., and THOMAS, L. A.: Study of chlamydiae in patients with lymphogranuloma venereum and urethritis attending a venereal disease clinic. Brit. J. vener. Dis. *47:* 114–121 (1971).

PHILIP, R. N.; LACKMAN, D. B.; FRANK, F. W.; MORRISON, J. D.; CASPER, E. A., and GREAVES, A. B.: Serologic reactions to specific complement-fixing antigens from microorganisms of the psittacosis-lymphogranuloma venereum-trachoma (PLT) group. Amer. J. Ophthal. *63:* 1499–1505 (1967).

POLLARD, M.: Ornithosis in sea-shore birds. Proc. Soc. exp. Biol. Med. *64:* 200–202 (1947).

POLLARD, M.; STARR, T. J.; TANAMI, Y., and MOORE, R. W.: Propagation of trachoma virus in cultures of human tissues. Proc. Soc. exp. Biol. Med. *104:* 223–225 (1960a).

POLLARD, M.; STARR, T. J.; MOORE, R. W., and TANAMI, Y.: Cytochemical changes in human amnion cells infected with psittacosis virus. Nature, Lond. *188:* 770 (1960b).

POLLARD, M. and TANAMI, Y.: Cytochemistry of trachoma virus replication in tissue cultures. Ann. N.Y. Acad. Sci. *98:* 50–61 (1962).

RAKE, G.: in BERGEY, MURRAY and HITCHES Manual of determinative bacteriology; 6th ed., pp. 1114–1120 (Williams & Wilkins, Baltimore 1957).

RAKE, G.; SHAFFER, M. F., and THYGESON, P.: Relationship of agents of trachoma and inclusion conjunctivitis to those of lymphogranuloma-psittacosis group. Proc. Soc. exp. Biol. Med. *49:* 545–547 (1942).

REEVE, P. and GRAHAM, D. M.: A neutralization test for trachoma and inclusion blennorrhoea viruses grown in HeLa cell cultures. J. gen. Microbiol. *27:* 177–180 (1962).

REEVE, P. and TAVERNE, J.: A simple method for total particle counts of trachoma and inclusion blennorrhea virus. Nature, Lond. *195:* 923–924 (1962).

REEVE, P. and TAVERNE, J.: Observations on the growth of trachoma and inclusion blennorrhea viruses in embryonated eggs. J. Hyg. *61:* 67–75 (1963).

REEVE, P. and TAVERNE, J.: The significance of strain differences in the behaviour of TRIC agents in the chick embryo. Amer. J. Ophthal. *63:* 1162–1166 (1967a).

REEVE, P. and TAVERNE, J.: An assessment of the evidence for regarding the T'ang strain as an authentic TRIC agent. Amer. J. Ophthal. *63:* 1437–1439 (1967b).

REEVE, P.; TAVERNE, J., and BUSHBY, S. R. M.: Inhibition by pyrimidine analogues of the synthesis of folic acid by trachoma agents. J. Hyg. *66:* 295–306 (1968).

RICE, C. E.: Carbohydrate matrix of the epithelial cell inclusion in trachoma. Proc. Soc. exp. Biol. Med. *33:* 317–318 (1935).

ROSENKRANZ, H. S.; GUTTER, B., and BECKER, Y.: Studies on the developmental cycle of *C. trachomatis.* Selective inhibition by hydroxyurea. J. Bact. *115:* 682–691 (1973).

ROSENKRANZ, H. S. and LEVY, J.: Hydroxyurea: a specific inhibitor of deoxyribonucleic acid synthesis. Biochim. biophys. Acta *95:* 181–183 (1965).

ROTA, T. R. and NICHOLS, R. L.: Infection of cell cultures by trachoma agent: enhancement by DEAE dextran. J. infect. Dis. *124:* 419–421 (1971).

SAROV, I. and BECKER, Y.: RNA in the elementary bodies of trachoma agent. Nature, Lond. *217:* 849–852 (1968).

SAROV, I. and BECKER, Y.: Trachoma agent DNA. J. molec. Biol. *42:* 581–589 (1969).

SAROV, I. and BECKER, Y.: DNA dependent RNA polymerase activity in purified trachoma elementary bodies. Effect of NaCl on RNA transcription. J. Bact. *107:*593–598 (1971a).

SAROV, I. and BECKER, Y.: DNA-dependent RNA polymerase in trachoma elementary bodies; in NICHOLS Trachoma and related disorders caused by chlamydial agents. Excerpta med. Int. Congr. Series No. 223, pp. 27–33 (1971b).

SCHACHTER, J.: A Bedsonia, isolated from a patient with clinical lymphogranuloma venereum. Amer. J. Ophthal. *63:* 1049–1053 (1967a).

SCHACHTER, J.: Isolation of Bedsoniae from human arthritis and abortion tissues. Amer. J. Ophthal. *63:* 1082–1086 (1967b).

SCHACHTER, J.: Complement-fixing antibodies to Bedsonia in Reiter's syndrome, TRIC agent infection and control groups. Amer. J. Ophthal. *71:* 857–860 (1971).

SHARON, N. and POLLARD, M.: Inhibition of T'ang trachoma agent by 5'-fluorodeoxycytidine. Proc. Soc. exp. Biol. Med. *114:* 344–347 (1963).

SHIAO, L. C.; WANG, S. P., and GRAYSTON, J. T.: Sensitivity and resistance of TRIC agents to penicillin, tetracycline and sulfa drugs. Amer. J. Ophthal. *63:* 1558–1568 (1967).

SHIH, A. Y.; EISENSTADT, J., and LENGYEL, P.: On the relation between ribonucleic acid synthesis and peptide chain initiation in *E. coli.* Proc. nat. Acad. Sci., Wash. *56:* 1599–1605 (1966).

SOWA, J. and RACE, M. W.: Sensitivity of trachoma agent to streptomycin and related antibiotics. J. Hyg. *69:* 709–716 (1971).

SOWA, S.; SOWA, J.; COLLIER, L. H., and BLYTH, V.: Trachoma and allied infections in a Gambian village. Medical Research Council, Special Report Series No. 308. HMSO London (1965).

SOWA, S.; SOWA, J.; COLLIER, L. H., and BLYTH, W. A.: Trachoma vaccine field trials in the Gambia. J. Hyg. *67:* 699–717 (1969).

STANIER, R. Y. and VAN NIEL, C. B.: The concept of a bacterium. Arch. Mikrobiol. *42:* 17–35 (1962).

STORZ, J.: Chlamydia and chlamydia-induced diseases (Thomas, Springfield 1971).

STORZ, J. and PAGE, L. A.: Taxonomy of the Chlamydiae: reasons for classifying organisms of the genus chlamydia family chlamydiaceae in a separate order chlamydiales ord. nov. Int. J. syst. Bact. *21:* 332–334 (1971).

TAJIMA, M.; NOMURA, Y., and KUBOTA, Y.: Structure and development of viruses of the psittacosis-lymphogranuloma group observed in the electron microscope. J. Bact. *74:* 605–620 (1957).

TAMURA, A.: Biochemical studies on the mechanism of infection of meningopneumonitis agent. Ann. Rep. Inst. Virus. Res. Kyoto *7:* 1–13 (1964a).

TAMURA, A.: Some properties of the trachoma agent grown in yolk sacs. J. all-India ophthal Soc. *12:* 59–64 (1964b).

TAMURA, A.: Isolation of ribosome particles from meningopneumonitis organisms. J. Bact. *93:* 2009–2016 (1967).

TAMURA, A. and IWANAGA, M.: RNA synthesis in cells infected with the meningopneumonitis agent. J. molec. Biol. *11:* 97–108 (1965).

T'ANG, F. F.; CHANG, H. L.; HUANG, Y. T., and WANG, K. C.: Studies on the etiology of trachoma with special reference to isolation of the virus in chick embryo. Chin. med. J. *75:* 429–447 (1957).

T'ANG, F. F.; HUANG, Y. T.; CHANG, H. L., and WANG, K. C.: Further studies on the isolation of trachoma virus. Acta virol., Prague *2:* 164–170 (1958).

TARIZZO, M. L.: Etudes sur le trachome. 1. Isolement et culture en série de 12 souches de virus sur œuf embryonné. Bull. Wld Hlth Org. *24:* 103–105 (1961).

TARIZZO, M. L. and NABLI, B.: The effect of antibiotics on the growth of TRIC agents in embryonated eggs. Amer. J. Ophthal. *63:* 1550–1557 (1967).

TARIZZO, M. L.; NABLI, B., and LABONNE, J.: Studies on trachoma. II. Evaluation of laboratory diagnostic methods under field conditions. Bull. Wld Hlth Org. *38:* 897–905 (1968).

TARIZZO, M. L. and NATAF, R.: The treatment of trachoma. Rev. int. Trach. *46:* 9–48 (1970).

TARIZZO, M. L. et NATAF, R.: Le traitement du trachome; dans PUIG et SOLANES Conc. 21st Ophthal., 1970. Excerpta med. Int. Congr. Series No. 222, pp. 1849–1875 (1971).

TAVERNE, J. and BLYTH, W. A.: Interactions between trachoma organisms and macrophages; in NICHOLS Trachoma and related disorders caused by chlamydial agents. Excerpta med. Int. Congr. Series No. 223, pp. 88–107 (1971).

TAVERNE, J.; BLYTH, W., and REEVE, P.: Toxicity of the agents of trachoma and inclusion conjunctivitis. J. gen. microbiol. *37:* 271–275 (1964).

TERSKIKH, I. I.; ZHDANOV, V. M., and BEKLESHOVA, H. IU.: Tkanevaia vakcina protiv trakhomy. I. Eksperimentalnoe isuchenie. Vop. Virus *9:* 275–279 (1964).

TERSKIKH, I. I.; ZHDANOV, V. M.; KUDOYAROV, R. G.; KUDOYAROV, G. H.; VORONTSOVA, Z. I.; MESHCHEROVA, N. K.; GROMYKO, A. I.; POPOVA, O. M., and YANBUCHTINA, F. A.: Vaccinotherapy and prophylaxis of relapses of trachoma. Rev. int. Trach. *44:* 201–217 (1967).

TERZIN, A. L.; VEDROS, N. A., and JOHNSTON, J. B.: Serological studies on group- and species-specific antigens of trachoma and inclusion conjunctivitis (TRIC) agents. J. Hyg. *62:* 185–198 (1964).

THYGESON, P.: Criteria of cure in trachoma with special reference to provocative tests. Rev. int. Trach. *30:* 450 (1953).

THYGESON, P.: Trachoma virus: historical background and review of isolates. Ann. N.Y. Acad. Sci. *98:* 6–13 (1962).

THYGESON, P.: Corneal changes in TRIC agent infections. Amer. J. Ophthal. *63:* 1278–1282 (1967).

TREHARNE, J. D.; KATZENELSON, E.; DAVEY, S. J., and GRAY, S. J.: Comparison of serotyping subgroup A chlamydial isolates by a one-way cross-reaction and by a two-way cross-reaction immunofluorescence test; in NICHOLS Trachoma and related disorders caused by chlamydial agents. Excerpta med. Int. Congr. Series No. 223, pp. 289–304 (1971).

TRIBBY, I. I. E.: Cell wall synthesis by *Chlamydia psittaci* growing in L cells. J. Bact. *104:* 1176–1188 (1970).

VILCEK, Y. and JAHIEL, R. I.: Action of interferon and its inducers against nonviral infectious agents. Arch. intern. Med. *126:* 69–77 (1970).

WANG, S. P.: A micro immunofluorescence method. Study of antibody response to TRIC organisms in mice; in NICHOLS Trachoma and related disorders caused by chlamydial agents. Excerpta med. Int. Congr. Series No. 223, pp. 273–288, (1971).

WANG, S. P. and GRAYSTON, J. T.: Pannus with experimental trachoma and inclusion conjunctivitis agent infection of Taiwan monkeys. Amer. J. Ophthal. *63:* 1133–1145 (1967a).

WANG, S. P. and GRAYSTON, J. T.: A potency test for trachoma vaccine utilizing the mouse toxicity prevention test. Amer. J. Ophthal *63:* 1443–1454 (1967b).

WANG, S. P. and GRAYSTON, J. T.: Immunological relationship between genital TRIC, lymphogranuloma venereum and related organisms in a new microtiter indirect immunofluorescence test. Amer. J. Ophthal. *70:* 367–374 (1970).

WANG, S. P. and GRAYSTON, J. T.: Studies on the identity of the 'fast' egg-killing chlamydia strains; in NICHOLS Trachoma and related disorders caused by chlamydial agents. Excerpta med. Int. Congr. Series No. 223, pp. 322–336 (1971a).

WANG, S. P. and GRAYSTON, J. T.: Local and systemic antibody response to trachoma eye infection in monkeys; in NICHOLS Trachoma and related disorders caused by chlamydial agents. Excerpta med. Int. Congr. Series No. 223, pp. 217–232 (1971b).

WANG, S. P. and GRAYSTON, J. T.: Classification of TRIC and related strains with micro-immunofluorescence; in NICHOLS Trachoma and related disorders caused by chlamydial agents. Excerpta med. Int. Congr. Series No. 223, pp. 305–321 (1971c).

WANG, S. P.; GRAYSTON, J. T., and ALEXANDER, E. R.: Trachoma vaccine studies in monkeys. Amer. J. Ophthal. *63:* 1615–1630 (1967a).

WANG, S. P.; GRAYSTON, J. T., and GALE, J. L.: Three new immunologic types of trachoma-inclusion conjunctivitis organisms, J. Immunol. *110:* 873–879 (1973).

WANG, S. P.; KENNY, G. E., and GRAYSTON, J. T.: Characterization of trachoma antigens protective against mouse toxicity. Amer. J. Ophthal. *63:* 1454–1461 (1967b).

WEHRLI, W. and STAEHELIN, M.: The rifamycins – relation to chemical structure and action on RNA polymerase. Biochim. biophys. Acta *182:* 24–29 (1969).

WEISS, E.: The nature of the psittacosis-lymphogranuloma group of microorganisms. Annu. Rev. Microbiol. *9:* 227–252 (1955).

WEISS, E.: Comparative metabolism of chlamydia with special reference to catabolic activities. Amer. J. Ophthal. *63:* 1098–1101 (1967a).

WEISS, E.: Transaminase activity and other enzymatic reactions involving pyruvate and glutamate in chlamydia (psittacosis-trachoma group). J. Bact. *93:* 177–184 (1967b).

WEISS, E.: Evolution of chlamydia; in NICHOLS Trachoma and related disorders caused by chlamydial agents. Excerpta med. Int. Congr. Series No. 223, pp. 3–12 (1971).

WEISS, E.; MYERS, W. F.; DRESSLER, H. R., and CHUN-HOON, H.: Glucose metabolism by agents of the psittacosis-trachoma group. Virology *22:* 551–562 (1964).

WEISS, E.; SCHRAMEK, S.; WILSON, N. N., and NEWMAN, L. W.: Deoxyribonucleic acid heterogeneity between human and murine strains of Chlamydia trachomatis. Infect. Immun. *2:* 24–28 (1970).

WEISBLUM, B. and DAVIES, J.: Antibiotic inhibitors of the bacterial ribosome. Bact. Rev. *32:* 493–528 (1968).

WENNER, H. A.: Psittacosis-lymphogranuloma group of viruses. Adv. virus Res. *5:* 39–93 (1958).

WERNER, G. H.: Recherches experimentales sur la chimothérapie du trachome. Ann. Inst. Pasteur *100:* 93–108 (1961).

WOOLRIDGE, R. L.; CHENG, K. H.; CHANG, I. H.; YANG, C. Y.; HSU, T. C., and GRAYSTON, J. T.: Failure of trachoma treatment with ophthalmic antibiotics and systemic sulfonamides used alone or in combination with trachoma vaccine. Amer. J. Ophthal *63:* 1577–1583 (1967a).

WOOLRIDGE, R. L.; GRAYSTON, J. T.; CHANG, I. H.; CHENG, K. H.; YANG, C. Y., and NEAVE, C.: Field trial of a monovalent and of a bivalent mineral oil adjuvant trachoma vaccine in Taiwan school children. Amer. J. Ophthal. *63:* 1645–1650 (1967b).

WOOLRIDGE, R. L.; GRAYSTON, J. T.; CHANG, I. H.; YANG, C. Y., and CHENG, K. H.: Long-term follow-up of the initial (1959–1960) trachoma vaccine field trial on Taiwan. Amer. J. Ophthal. *63:* 1650–1653 (1967c).

ZAKAY-RONES, Z. and BECKER, Y.: Antibodies to trachoma elementary bodies; in NICHOLS Trachoma and related disorders caused by chlamydial agents. Excerpta med. Int. Congr. Series No. 223, pp. 254–259 (1971).

ZAKAY-RONES, Z.; KATZENELSON, E., and LEVY, R.: Hemagglutinin of trachoma agent. Israel J. med. Sci. *4:* 305–306 (1968).

ZAKAY-RONES, Z.; LEVI, R.; MAYTHAR, B., and BECKER, Y.: The antibody response of guinea pigs to topical and intramuscular administration of trachoma antigens. J. Immunol. *102:* 1290–1294 (1969).

